KIDNEY STONE DIET COOKBOOK FOR BEGINNERS: Essential recipes for stone kidney management

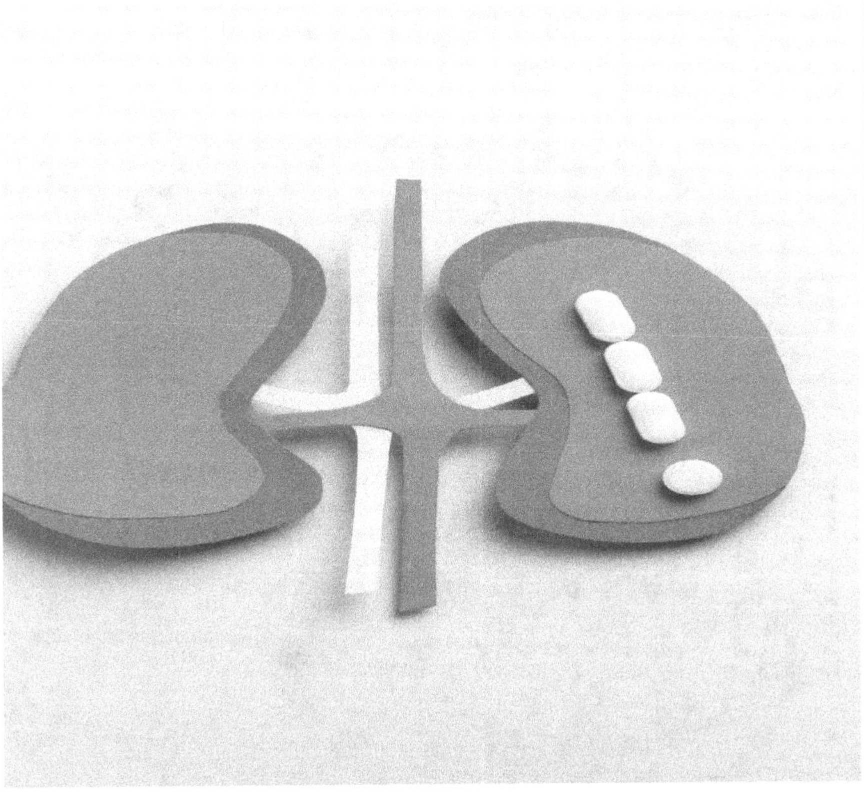

ETHEL D. AYER

rights reserved. No part of this publication may be reproduced, distributed, or transmitted in any form or by any means, including photocopying, recording, or other electronic or mechanical methods, without the prior written permission of the publisher, except in the case of brief quotations embodied in critical reviews and certain other non-commercial uses permitted by copyright law.

Copyright © , ETHEL D. AYER, 2024.

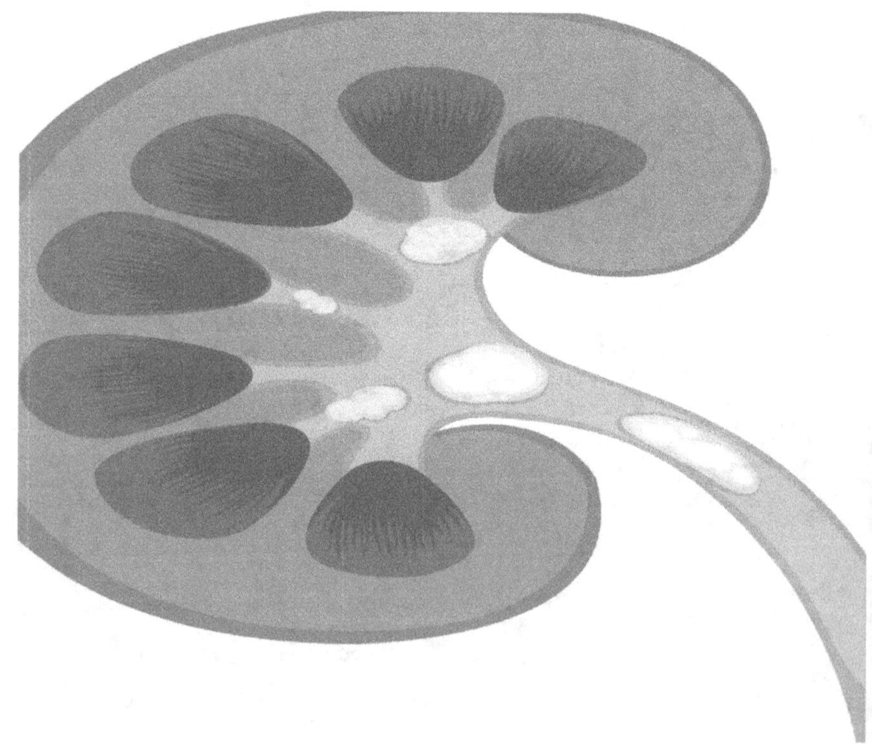

INTRODUCTION

Once upon a time in a quaint little town nestled between rolling hills, there lived a woman named Emily. Emily was a bubbly soul who loved nothing more than indulging in delicious foods from around the world. However, her joy was abruptly interrupted when she was diagnosed with kidney stones.

Faced with excruciating pain and discomfort, Emily's doctor recommended a strict kidney stone diet to prevent further complications. Determined to reclaim her health and vitality, Emily embarked on a journey to explore the world of kidney-friendly cuisine.

Armed with determination and a thirst for knowledge, Emily stumbled upon a hidden gem – a kidney stone diet cookbook for beginners. With its vibrant cover and promises of delicious, stone-free meals, Emily couldn't resist giving it a try.

As she flipped through the pages, Emily was delighted to find a plethora of mouthwatering recipes tailored specifically for those with kidney stones. From flavorful salads bursting with fresh veggies to hearty soups brimming with nourishing ingredients, the cookbook offered a treasure trove of culinary delights.

Eager to put her newfound knowledge to the test, Emily ventured into the kitchen with gusto. Armed with pots, pans, and an array of kidney-friendly ingredients, she set to work creating her first recipe – a tantalizing quinoa salad with roasted vegetables.

As the aroma of herbs and spices filled the air, Emily couldn't help but feel a sense of anticipation building within her. With each bite of the delicious salad, she savored the flavors and textures, knowing that she was nourishing her body from the inside out.

Weeks turned into months, and Emily diligently continued to explore the recipes within the kidney stone diet cookbook. With each passing day, she noticed a remarkable improvement in her health and well-being. The once unbearable pain of kidney stones became a distant memory, replaced by a newfound sense of vitality and energy.

Word of Emily's remarkable transformation spread throughout the town, inspiring others who were struggling with similar health issues to embark on their own journey to wellness.

Before long, the kidney stone diet cookbook became a bestseller, touching the lives of countless individuals seeking relief from the burden of kidney stones.

As Emily reflected on her journey, she couldn't help but feel grateful for the unexpected gift that had come into her life. Through the pages of a simple cookbook, she had discovered not only the power of food to heal but also the strength of the human spirit to overcome adversity.

And so, with a heart full of gratitude and a newfound zest for life, Emily continued her stone-free journey, embracing each day with renewed passion and purpose. For in the pages of a cookbook, she had found not only recipes for nourishing meals but also the ingredients for a life filled with health, happiness, and endless possibilities.

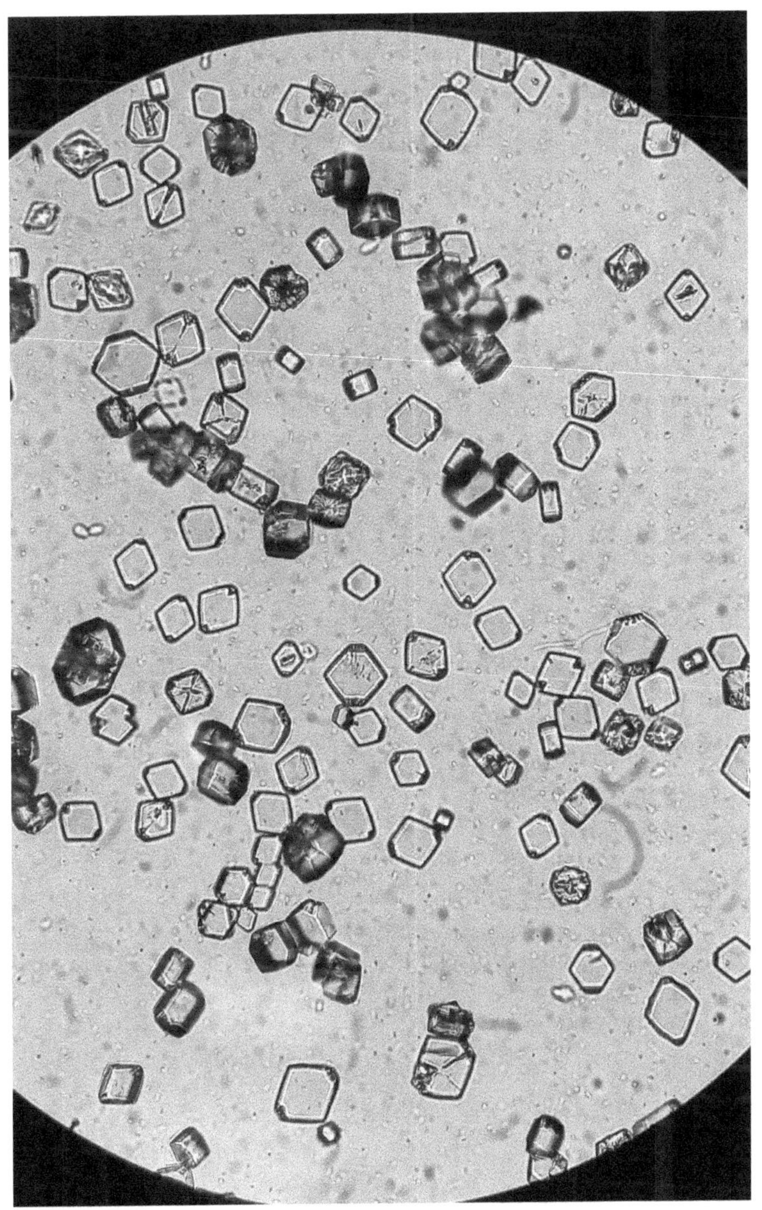

CHAPTER 1: UNDERSTANDING KIDNEY STONES

Types of Kidney Stones

Kidney stones, though small, can bring immense pain and discomfort. Understanding the different types of kidney stones is crucial for proper treatment and prevention.

Calcium Stones:

These are the most common type, comprising calcium oxalate or calcium phosphate. Excess calcium in the urine combines with other substances like oxalate, forming solid crystals that can grow into stones.

- **Struvite Stones:** Also known as infection stones, these form in response to urinary tract infections (UTIs). They can grow quickly and become quite large, often requiring medical intervention for removal.

- **Uric Acid Stones:** When the urine is too acidic, uric acid crystals can form, leading to stones. Factors like a high-protein diet or certain medical conditions can contribute to their formation.

- **Cystine Stones:** These are rare and occur in people with a hereditary disorder called cystinuria. It causes the kidneys to excrete excessive amounts of certain amino acids, leading to stone formation.
- Other Stones: Less common types include xanthine stones (related to a genetic disorder) and drug-induced stones (caused by certain medications).

Causes and Risk Factors

- Kidney stones develop when certain substances in the urine, such as calcium, oxalate, and uric acid, become highly concentrated and form crystals. These crystals can then aggregate and develop into stones. Several factors contribute to the formation of kidney stones:

- **Dehydration:** Inadequate fluid intake reduces urine volume, allowing minerals and salts to become more concentrated and facilitating stone formation.

- **Diet:** Consuming foods high in oxalate, sodium, or protein can increase the risk of kidney stones. Oxalate-rich foods include spinach, nuts, and chocolate, while excessive sodium intake can lead to higher calcium levels in the urine, promoting stone formation.

- **Family or Personal History:** A family history of kidney stones increases the likelihood of developing them. Additionally, individuals who have previously experienced kidney stones are at higher risk of recurrence.

- **Medical Conditions: Certain medical conditions, such as obesity, diabetes**, high blood pressure, and digestive disorders, can increase the risk of kidney stones. People with specific metabolic disorders, like hyperparathyroidism or cystinuria, are also more prone to stone formation.

- **Lifestyle Factors:** Sedentary lifestyle habits, as well as certain occupations that involve prolonged periods of sitting or dehydration, can contribute to kidney stone development.

Importance of Dietary Management

Dietary management plays a crucial role in preventing the formation and recurrence of kidney stones. Here's why it's so important:

- **Control Mineral Intake:** Certain minerals like calcium, oxalate, and sodium can contribute to kidney stone formation. By adjusting the intake of foods rich in these minerals, individuals can reduce the risk of stone development.

- For example, consuming calcium-rich foods alongside oxalate-rich foods can help prevent oxalate from binding with calcium in the urine, thus reducing the formation of calcium oxalate stones.

- **Maintain Proper Hydration:** Adequate fluid intake is essential for diluting urine and preventing the concentration of minerals that can lead to stone formation. Drinking plenty of water throughout the day helps flush out minerals and prevents them from crystallizing in the kidneys.

- **Limit Certain Foods:** Some foods, such as high-oxalate foods like spinach and nuts, or high-sodium foods like processed meats and canned soups, can increase the risk of kidney stones.
- Dietary management involves limiting the consumption of these foods to maintain optimal urinary health.

- **Promote Overall Health:** A kidney stone diet emphasizes whole foods, fruits, vegetables, and lean proteins, which not only help prevent stone formation but also promote overall health.

By following a balanced and nutritious diet, individuals can support their kidney function and reduce the risk of developing other health conditions associated with poor dietary habits.

The Kidney Stone Diet Basics

❖ **Key Principles of the Diet**

The diet for kidney stone prevention revolves around several key principles aimed at reducing the risk of stone formation and promoting urinary health:

- **Hydration:** Adequate fluid intake is essential to maintain urine dilution and prevent the concentration of minerals that can form stones. Water is the preferred beverage, and individuals are encouraged to drink enough to produce at least 2 liters of urine per day.

- **Balanced Calcium Intake:** Contrary to popular belief, consuming adequate calcium from foods like dairy products can actually help prevent kidney stone formation by binding with oxalate in the intestines, preventing it from being absorbed into the bloodstream and excreted in the urine.

- **Moderate Oxalate Intake:** While some high-oxalate foods like spinach and almonds can contribute to stone formation, it's not necessary to completely eliminate them from the diet. Instead, individuals are advised to consume these foods in moderation and pair them with calcium-rich foods to reduce the risk of oxalate absorption.

- **Limit Sodium and Protein:** Excessive sodium and protein intake can increase urinary calcium excretion, leading to higher stone formation risk. Therefore, it's important to limit the consumption of salty foods and opt for lean protein sources.

- **Maintain a Healthy Weight:** Obesity is a risk factor for kidney stones, so maintaining a healthy weight through a balanced diet and regular physical activity can help reduce the likelihood of stone formation.

Hydration and Its Role

Hydration plays a pivotal role in kidney stone prevention and management due to its impact on urine volume and composition. Here's how hydration affects kidney stone formation:

- **Dilution of Minerals:** Adequate hydration ensures that urine remains diluted, reducing the concentration of minerals like calcium, oxalate, and uric acid.

  When these minerals are present in high concentrations, they are more likely to crystallize and form stones. Drinking plenty of water helps keep urine volume high, making it less likely for minerals to precipitate and form crystals.

- **Promotion of Urinary Flow:** Proper hydration facilitates the flow of urine through the urinary tract, preventing the stagnation of urine and the buildup of minerals that can lead to stone formation. Increased urine flow helps flush out crystals and small stones before they have a chance to grow larger and cause obstruction or pain.

- **Prevention of Stone Recurrence:** For individuals who have previously experienced kidney stones, maintaining adequate hydration is crucial for preventing recurrence. By consistently drinking enough water each day, individuals can minimize the risk of stone formation and reduce the likelihood of experiencing another painful episode.

- **Choice of Beverage:** While water is the best choice for hydration, other beverages such as herbal teas and diluted fruit juices can also contribute to fluid intake. However, it's important to avoid excessive consumption of sugary or caffeinated beverages, as these can have negative effects on urinary health.

Balancing Nutrients

Balancing nutrients is crucial for kidney stone prevention as it helps maintain optimal urinary health and reduces the risk of stone formation. Here's how balancing nutrients plays a key role:

- **Calcium:** Contrary to popular belief, adequate calcium intake is essential for kidney stone prevention. Calcium binds with oxalate in the intestines, reducing its absorption and lowering the risk of calcium oxalate stone formation. However, it's important to obtain calcium from dietary sources rather than supplements, and to consume it in conjunction with oxalate-containing foods for optimal absorption.

- **Oxalate:** While oxalate is naturally present in many foods, excessive intake can contribute to calcium oxalate stone formation. Balancing oxalate intake with calcium-rich foods helps prevent oxalate from binding with calcium in the urinary tract and forming stones. High-oxalate foods like spinach, nuts, and chocolate should be consumed in moderation, especially for individuals at higher risk of stone formation.

- **Sodium:** Excessive sodium intake can increase urinary calcium excretion, leading to higher stone formation risk. Balancing sodium intake by reducing consumption of processed and salty foods helps maintain urinary calcium levels within a healthy range and reduces the risk of stone formation.

- **Protein:** High-protein diets can increase urinary excretion of calcium and uric acid, potentially increasing the risk of kidney stone formation. Balancing protein intake by choosing lean protein sources and moderating consumption helps prevent excessive urinary excretion of stone-forming substances.

CHAPTER 2: BUILDING A KIDNEY-FRIENDLY KITCHEN

Stocking the Pantry

❖ Essential Ingredients

Essential ingredients for a kidney stone diet focus on promoting urinary health, preventing stone formation, and supporting overall well-being. Here are some key ingredients to include:

- **Water:** Adequate hydration is essential for maintaining urine dilution and preventing the concentration of minerals that can lead to stone formation. Drinking plenty of water throughout the day helps flush out minerals and toxins from the urinary tract, reducing the risk of stone development.

- **Calcium-Rich Foods:** Contrary to common misconceptions, consuming calcium-rich foods is important for preventing kidney stones. Calcium binds with oxalate in the intestines, preventing its absorption and reducing the risk of calcium oxalate stone formation. Incorporating sources like dairy products, leafy greens, and fortified foods can help ensure adequate calcium intake.

- **Low-Oxalate Foods:** While oxalate is naturally present in many foods, excessive intake can contribute to stone formation. Including low-oxalate options like cauliflower, cabbage, and berries in the diet can help reduce the risk of calcium oxalate stone formation.

- **Fruits and Vegetables:** Fruits and vegetables are rich in vitamins, minerals, and antioxidants that support overall health and urinary tract function. Additionally, their high water content helps promote hydration and urine dilution, reducing the risk of stone formation.

- **Lean Protein Sources:** Opting for lean protein sources like poultry, fish, and legumes helps maintain a balanced diet while reducing the risk of excessive urinary excretion of stone-forming substances like calcium and uric acid.

Substitutes for High-Risk Foods

Substituting high-risk foods with healthier alternatives is a key strategy for reducing the risk of kidney stone formation. Here are some substitutions for common high-risk foods:

- **High-Oxalate Foods:** Instead of spinach, opt for kale or Swiss chard, which are lower in oxalate content.
  Substitute almonds and peanuts with pistachios or cashews, which have lower oxalate levels.
  Choose white rice or quinoa over brown rice, as it contains less oxalate.

- **High-Sodium Foods:** Replace processed meats like bacon and sausage with lean cuts of poultry or fish.
  Use fresh herbs, spices, and citrus juices to season foods instead of salt.
  Opt for low-sodium or sodium-free versions of canned soups, broths, and sauces.

- **High-Protein Foods:** Incorporate plant-based protein sources like tofu, tempeh, and legumes into meals.

Choose lean cuts of meat like chicken or turkey breast instead of fatty cuts or processed meats.
Limit intake of high-protein foods like red meat and organ meats, opting for moderation instead.

- **High-Sugar Foods:** Substitute sugary beverages with water, herbal teas, or infused water with fruits or herbs.
Choose fresh fruits or unsweetened dried fruits as snacks instead of sugary snacks or candies.
Use natural sweeteners like honey or maple syrup in moderation instead of refined sugars.

- **Reading Food Labels:** Reading food labels is essential for individuals seeking to prevent kidney stone formation by making informed dietary choices. Here's why it's important and how to do it effectively:

- **Identify High-Risk Ingredients:** Food labels provide valuable information about the nutritional content of products, including the presence of high-risk ingredients like oxalate, sodium, and added sugars. By carefully reading labels, individuals can identify foods that may increase the risk of kidney stone formation and make healthier choices.

- **Check Serving Sizes:** Paying attention to serving sizes is crucial for accurately assessing nutrient content. Some foods may appear low in certain nutrients per serving, but consuming larger portions can lead to higher intake levels. By comparing serving sizes and adjusting portions accordingly, individuals can better manage their nutrient intake and reduce the risk of stone formation.

- **Look for Low-Risk Options:** When shopping for foods, prioritize options that are low in oxalate, sodium, and added sugars. Choosing whole, unprocessed foods like fruits, vegetables, lean proteins, and whole grains can help support kidney health and reduce the risk of stone formation.

- **Be Mindful of Hidden Ingredients:** Some foods may contain hidden ingredients that can contribute to kidney stone formation, such as preservatives, artificial sweeteners, and flavor enhancers. Reading food labels carefully can help individuals identify these ingredients and make more informed choices about their dietary intake.

❖ **Kitchen Tools and Techniques**
Cooking Methods that Preserve Nutrients
Cooking methods that preserve nutrients are beneficial for individuals seeking to maintain a kidney stone diet while maximizing nutritional intake. Here are some cooking techniques that help retain essential nutrients:

- **Steaming:** Steaming is a gentle cooking method that involves using steam to cook food without submerging it in water. This technique helps preserve the natural flavors, colors, and nutrients of fruits, vegetables, and lean proteins. Steamed vegetables like broccoli, carrots, and cauliflower retain their crisp texture and nutrient content, making them ideal choices for a kidney stone diet.

- **Grilling or Broiling:** Grilling or broiling food over an open flame or direct heat source allows for quick cooking while retaining nutrients. Lean proteins like chicken breast, fish fillets, and tofu can be grilled or broiled to perfection, locking in moisture and flavor without the need for excessive added fats.

- **Stir-Frying:** Stir-frying involves cooking food quickly over high heat in a small amount of oil. This method preserves the texture and nutrients of vegetables, proteins, and whole grains while imparting delicious flavors. Stir-fried dishes with colorful vegetables and lean proteins like shrimp or tofu provide a nutritious and kidney stone-friendly meal option.

- **Raw Preparation:** Opting for raw preparations like salads, crudité platters, and fresh fruit bowls allows for maximum retention of vitamins, minerals, and enzymes. Raw fruits and vegetables are rich in water and fiber, making them hydrating and nourishing choices for individuals following a kidney stone diet.

- **Portion Control Tips**
Portion control is essential for individuals managing kidney stones, as excessive intake of certain nutrients can increase the risk of

stone formation. Here are some portion control tips for a kidney stone diet:

- **Use Smaller Plates:** Opting for smaller plates and bowls can help control portion sizes by visually tricking the brain into thinking there is more food present. This can prevent overeating and promote healthier portion sizes.

- **Measure Servings:** Use measuring cups, spoons, or kitchen scales to accurately portion out foods, especially high-risk items like nuts, seeds, and dried fruits. This ensures that servings are in line with recommended intake levels and helps prevent excessive consumption of nutrients like oxalate and sodium.

- **Fill Half Your Plate with Vegetables:** Vegetables are low in calories and high in fiber, vitamins, and minerals, making them ideal for filling up without consuming excessive calories or nutrients that may contribute to stone formation. Aim to fill at least half of your plate with non-starchy vegetables like leafy greens, peppers, and cucumbers.

- **Practice Mindful Eating:** Pay attention to hunger and fullness cues, and eat slowly to savor each bite. This allows time for the brain to register feelings of fullness, reducing the likelihood of overeating. Avoid distractions like television or screens while eating to focus on the meal and prevent mindless snacking.

- **Be Aware of Restaurant Portions:** Restaurant portions are often larger than necessary, so consider sharing entrees or asking for a half portion. Alternatively, request a to-go container upfront and portion out a sensible serving size before starting your meal.

Meal Preparation Strategies

Meal preparation is a valuable strategy for individuals managing kidney stones, as it allows for careful control of ingredients, portions, and cooking methods. Here are some meal preparation strategies tailored to a kidney stone diet:

- **Plan Balanced Meals:** Plan meals that include a balance of lean proteins, healthy fats, whole grains, and plenty of fruits and vegetables. Aim to include a variety of colors and textures to maximize nutrient intake and support overall health.

- **Incorporate Low-Risk Foods:** Prioritize foods that are low in oxalate, sodium, and added sugars, as these nutrients can contribute to stone formation. Include plenty of hydrating fruits and vegetables like cucumbers, watermelon, and bell peppers, as well as lean proteins like chicken, fish, and tofu.

- **Batch Cook Protein Sources:** Prepare lean protein sources like grilled chicken breast, baked fish fillets, or marinated tofu in large batches and portion them out for use throughout the week. This saves time and ensures that nutritious protein options are readily available for meals and snacks.

- **Pre-Cut Vegetables and Fruits:** Wash, chop, and pre-portion vegetables and fruits for quick and convenient snacking or meal additions. Having pre-cut produce on hand makes it easier to incorporate healthy choices into meals and reduces the temptation to reach for less nutritious options.

- **Choose Kidney-Friendly Cooking Methods:** Opt for cooking methods that preserve nutrients and minimize the use of added fats and salts. Steaming, grilling, broiling, and stir-frying are excellent options that retain the natural flavors and textures of foods while minimizing the risk of stone formation.

- **Portion Control:** Use smaller plates and measuring tools to control portion sizes and prevent overeating. Be mindful of recommended serving sizes for high-risk foods like nuts, seeds, and dairy products, and practice moderation to avoid excessive intake of nutrients that may contribute to stone formation.

- **Pack Balanced Lunches:** Prepare balanced lunches ahead of time by packing a combination of protein, whole grains, fruits, and vegetables in reusable containers.

This ensures that nutritious options are readily available for busy days and helps prevent the temptation to rely on convenience foods that may be less kidney-friendly.

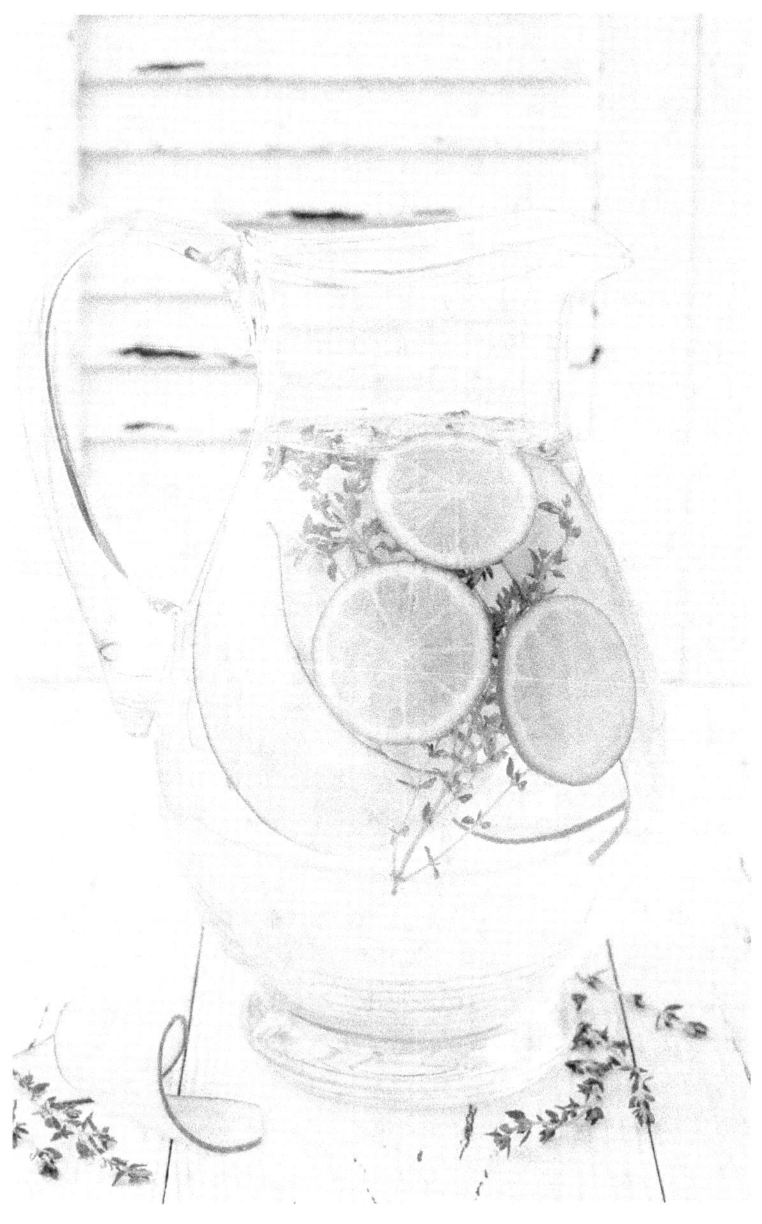

CHAPTER 3: HYDRATION HABITS

The Power of Water

❖ Optimal Daily Water Intake

Optimal daily water intake is crucial for kidney stone prevention, as it helps maintain urine dilution and reduces the concentration of minerals that can form stones.

The recommended daily water intake varies depending on factors such as age, weight, activity level, climate, and overall health status.

However, a general guideline for kidney stone prevention is to aim for at least 2 to 3 liters (about 8 to 12 cups) of fluid per day.

For individuals with a history of kidney stones or at higher risk of stone formation, healthcare providers may recommend higher fluid intake to ensure adequate hydration.

Some experts suggest aiming for urine output of about 2.5 to 3 liters per day to reduce the risk of stone recurrence effectively.

Water is the best choice for hydration, but other fluids like herbal teas, diluted fruit juices, and broths can also contribute to total fluid intake.

However, it's essential to avoid excessive consumption of sugary or caffeinated beverages, as they can have negative effects on urinary health.

Staying well-hydrated throughout the day, maintaining clear or light yellow urine color, and monitoring fluid intake are essential strategies for kidney stone prevention.

By meeting optimal daily water intake recommendations, individuals can support urinary health, prevent stone formation, and reduce the risk of stone recurrence.

Creative Ways to Stay Hydrated

Staying hydrated is essential for kidney stone prevention, but it can sometimes be challenging to meet daily fluid intake goals.

Here are some creative ways to stay hydrated and make it easier to reach optimal fluid intake levels:

- **Flavor Infusions:** Infuse water with fresh fruits, vegetables, or herbs to add flavor and variety. Citrus slices, cucumber, mint, berries, and ginger are excellent options for enhancing the taste of water without adding calories or sugar.

- **Herbal Teas:** Enjoy a variety of herbal teas throughout the day to increase fluid intake while providing warmth and comfort. Choose caffeine-free options like chamomile, peppermint, or rooibos for optimal hydration without the diuretic effects of caffeine.

- **Hydration Apps:** Use smartphone apps or wearable devices to track fluid intake and set reminders to drink water regularly. These apps can help you stay accountable and ensure you're meeting daily hydration goals.

- **Hydrating Foods:** Incorporate hydrating foods like watermelon, cucumber, celery, oranges, and strawberries into meals and snacks. These foods have high water content and contribute to total fluid intake w
hile providing essential nutrients and fiber.

- **Sip Throughout the Day:** Carry a reusable water bottle with you wherever you go and take sips regularly throughout the day. Setting specific times to drink water, such as upon waking, before meals, and during breaks, can help establish a hydration routine.

- **Sparkling Water:** Enjoy sparkling water or carbonated water as an alternative to plain water for a refreshing and bubbly beverage option. Look for varieties without added sugars or artificial sweeteners for optimal hydration.

Herbal Teas and Infusions

Herbal teas and infusions can be valuable additions to a kidney stone diet, offering hydration and potential health benefits without the risk of contributing to stone formation. Here are some herbal teas and infusions that may be beneficial for kidney stone prevention:

- **Dandelion Tea:** Dandelion root tea is believed to have diuretic properties, promoting increased urine production and helping flush out toxins and waste from the kidneys. It may also support liver function and aid in digestion.

- **Nettle Tea:** Nettle leaf tea is thought to have mild diuretic effects and may help reduce inflammation in the urinary tract. It is rich in vitamins, minerals, and antioxidants, making it a nourishing option for overall kidney health.

- **Corn Silk Tea:** Corn silk tea is made from the silky threads found on corn ears and is believed to have diuretic properties that support kidney function and promote urine flow. It may also help reduce urinary tract inflammation and irritation.

- **Hibiscus Tea:** Hibiscus tea is rich in antioxidants and has been shown to have potential benefits for kidney health. It may help lower blood pressure and reduce the risk of kidney stones by inhibiting the formation of calcium oxalate crystals.

- **Lemongrass Infusion:** Lemongrass is known for its mild diuretic properties and may help increase urine production, promoting kidney function and flushing out toxins. It also adds a refreshing citrusy flavor to beverages.

Beverages to Limit or Avoid

❖ **High Oxalate and Phosphate Beverages**
High oxalate and phosphate beverages should be consumed with caution by individuals prone to kidney stones, as these compounds can contribute to stone formation. Here are some examples of beverages containing high levels of oxalate and phosphate:

- **Dark Beer:** Dark beers like stout and porter contain higher levels of oxalate compared to lighter beer varieties. Oxalate is a naturally occurring compound found in barley, a key ingredient in beer production.

- **Chocolate Milk:** Chocolate milk contains both oxalate and phosphate, with higher levels found in cocoa powder and chocolate flavorings. While milk itself is a good source of calcium, which can help prevent oxalate absorption, the added oxalate and phosphate content in chocolate milk should be considered for those at risk of kidney stones.

- **Colas and Soda:** Colas and other carbonated sodas are high in phosphate, which can contribute to the formation of calcium phosphate stones. Additionally, some sodas contain added oxalate in the form of phosphoric acid, further increasing the risk of stone formation.

- **Almond Milk:** Almond milk can be high in oxalate, especially when fortified with calcium carbonate, which is often used to increase its calcium content. While almond milk is generally lower in oxalate compared to other nut-based beverages, individuals prone to kidney stones should be mindful of their intake.

Sugary Drinks and Their Impact

Sugary drinks can have a significant impact on kidney stone formation and overall urinary health. Here's how:

- **Increased Oxalate Excretion:** High consumption of sugary drinks, particularly those containing fructose, can lead to increased urinary oxalate excretion. Excessive oxalate in the urine can combine with calcium to form calcium oxalate stones, the most common type of kidney stone.

- **Dehydration:** Sugary drinks like soda, sports drinks, and sweetened fruit juices often contain caffeine, which has diuretic properties that can increase urine output and lead to dehydration. Dehydration can result in more concentrated urine, promoting the crystallization of minerals and increasing the risk of stone formation

- **Acidic Environment:** Many sugary drinks are acidic, with a low pH level that can contribute to the formation of uric acid stones. The acidic environment in the urine can lead to the precipitation of uric acid crystals, which can grow into stones over time.

- **Weight Gain and Obesity:** Regular consumption of sugary drinks is associated with weight gain and obesity, both of which are risk factors for kidney stone formation. Excess body weight can lead to changes in urinary chemistry and increase the likelihood of stone development.

CHAPTER 4: BREAKFASTS FOR KIDNEY HEALTH

Protein-Packed Breakfasts

❖ Lean Protein Choices

When considering lean protein choices for kidney stone prevention or management, it's crucial to focus on options that are low in purines and oxalates, as these substances can contribute to the formation of certain types of kidney stones. Here are some excellent lean protein choices to include in your diet:

- **Poultry:** Skinless chicken and turkey are excellent sources of lean protein that are generally low in purines. Opt for white meat over dark meat to keep purine intake minimal.

- **Fish:** Many types of fish, such as salmon, trout, and tuna, are not only rich in lean protein but also provide omega-3 fatty acids, which have anti-inflammatory properties and may help reduce the risk of kidney stone formation.

- **Legumes:** Beans, lentils, and peas are plant-based sources of lean protein that are also high in fiber, which can help prevent the formation of kidney stones by promoting regular bowel movements and reducing the absorption of oxalates.

- **Eggs:** Eggs are a versatile and affordable source of lean protein. While they contain purines, they are generally considered safe in moderation for most people, especially when consumed as part of a balanced diet.

- **Low-fat dairy:** Dairy products like milk, yogurt, and cheese can be excellent sources of lean protein, calcium, and vitamin D. Opt for low-fat or fat-free varieties to minimize saturated fat intake.

Egg Variations

When considering egg variations for kidney stone prevention or management, it's essential to balance the intake of purines and oxalates, which can contribute to the formation of certain types of kidney stones. Here are some egg variations to consider:

- **Egg Whites:** Egg whites are a lean source of protein that are virtually free of purines and low in oxalates. They provide the protein your body needs without adding to the risk of kidney stone formation.

- **Boiled Eggs:** Hard-boiled eggs are a convenient and versatile option that can be enjoyed as a snack or added to salads and sandwiches. Boiling eggs doesn't significantly alter their purine or oxalate content, making them a safe choice for individuals at risk of kidney stones.

- **Omelets with Low-Oxalate Ingredients:** Incorporating vegetables such as bell peppers, mushrooms, and spinach into your omelets can add flavor and nutrients without significantly increasing oxalate intake. These ingredients also provide fiber, vitamins, and minerals that support overall kidney health.

- **Egg Substitutes:** For those looking to reduce egg consumption or avoid dietary cholesterol, egg substitutes made from egg whites or plant-based ingredients can be a suitable alternative. Many egg substitutes are low in purines and oxalates, making them kidney stone-friendly options.

- **Moderation and Balance:** While eggs can be part of a kidney stone-friendly diet, it's essential to consume them in moderation and alongside other low-purine and low-oxalate foods. Maintaining a balanced diet that includes a variety of nutrient-dense foods is key to preventing kidney stones and supporting overall health.

Plant-Based Protein Options

Plant-based protein options can be excellent choices for individuals seeking to prevent kidney stones, as many plant-based foods are low in purines and oxalates while being rich in essential nutrients and fiber. Here are some plant-based protein options to consider:

- **Legumes:** Beans, lentils, and peas are excellent sources of plant-based protein that are low in purines and oxalates. They are also high in fiber, which can help prevent the formation of kidney stones by promoting regular bowel movements and reducing the absorption of oxalates.

- **Tofu and Tempeh:** Soy-based products like tofu and tempeh are versatile plant-based protein options that can be used in a variety of dishes. They are low in purines and oxalates and provide essential amino acids necessary for overall health.

- **Nuts and Seeds:** Almonds, walnuts, chia seeds, and hemp seeds are nutrient-dense sources of plant-based protein that are also low in purines and oxalates. They are rich in healthy fats, fiber, vitamins, and minerals, making them a valuable addition to a kidney stone-friendly diet.

- **Quinoa:** Quinoa is a gluten-free whole grain that is high in protein and low in purines and oxalates. It's also a good source of fiber, iron, magnesium, and other essential nutrients, making it an excellent choice for individuals looking to support kidney health.

- **Plant-Based Protein Powders:** Pea protein, rice protein, and hemp protein powders are popular plant-based protein supplements that can be added to smoothies, oatmeal, or baked goods. They offer a convenient way to increase protein intake without adding significant amounts of purines or oxalates to the diet.

Grain and Cereal Alternatives

❖ **Low-Oxalate Grains**

Low-oxalate grains are an important component of a kidney stone-friendly diet, especially for individuals prone to calcium oxalate stones. Here are some low-oxalate grains to consider incorporating into your meals:

- **Rice:** White rice, brown rice, and wild rice are all low-oxalate grains that can serve as versatile and filling staples in your diet. They can be used as a base for stir-fries, pilafs, salads, or served alongside protein and vegetables.

- **Oats:** Oats are a nutritious whole grain that is naturally low in oxalates. They are high in fiber, which can help promote regular bowel movements and reduce the absorption of oxalates in the gut. Enjoy oatmeal for breakfast or use oats in baking recipes for added texture and nutrition.

- **Barley:** Barley is a hearty and flavorful grain that is low in oxalates and rich in fiber, vitamins, and minerals. It can be used in soups, stews, salads, or as a side dish similar to rice or quinoa.

- **Millet:** Millet is a gluten-free grain that is low in oxalates and easy to digest. It has a mild flavor and a slightly crunchy texture, making it a versatile ingredient for both sweet and savory dishes.

- **Buckwheat:** Despite its name, buckwheat is not related to wheat and is naturally low in oxalates. It can be used to make gluten-free pancakes, porridge, or added to salads and stir-fries for a nutritious boost.

Homemade Granola and Muesli

Homemade granola and muesli can be excellent additions to a kidney stone-friendly diet, as they allow you to control the ingredients and ensure they are low in oxalates and high in nutrient-rich components. Here's how you can create kidney stone-friendly versions of these beloved breakfast options:

- **Choose Low-Oxalate Grains:** Opt for grains such as oats, rice flakes, or puffed rice as the base of your homemade granola or muesli. These grains are low in oxalates and provide fiber, which can help promote regular bowel movements and reduce the absorption of oxalates in the gut.

- **Include Nutrient-Dense Nuts and Seeds:** Add a variety of nuts and seeds to your granola or muesli for extra protein, healthy fats, vitamins, and minerals. Almonds, walnuts, pumpkin seeds, and sunflower seeds are excellent choices that are low in oxalates and rich in nutrients.

- **Limit High-Oxalate Ingredients:** Be cautious with ingredients such as almonds and cashews, which are higher in oxalates compared to other nuts. Use them sparingly or choose alternatives that are lower in oxalates, such as pecans or pistachios.

- **Sweeten Wisely:** Use natural sweeteners like honey, maple syrup, or agave nectar in moderation to add sweetness to your granola or muesli. Avoid using processed sugars or artificial sweeteners, which can have negative effects on overall health.

- **Customize with Fruit:** Incorporate dried fruits such as raisins, cranberries, or apricots into your granola or muesli for added flavor and sweetness. While some fruits contain moderate levels of oxalates, they can still be enjoyed in moderation as part of a balanced diet.

Breakfast Smoothies

Breakfast smoothies can be a delicious and convenient way to start your day while supporting kidney stone prevention or management. By choosing the right ingredients, you can create smoothies that are low in oxalates and rich in nutrients that promote kidney health. Here's how:

- **Base:** Start with a liquid base such as water, coconut water, almond milk, or low-fat dairy milk. These options are generally low in oxalates and provide hydration without adding excessive calories or sugar.

- **Low-Oxalate Fruits:** Incorporate fruits that are low in oxalates into your smoothie, such as berries (e.g., strawberries, blueberries, raspberries), melons, peaches, or bananas. These fruits provide natural sweetness, fiber, and essential vitamins and minerals without contributing to kidney stone formation.

- **Leafy Greens:** Add a handful of leafy greens like spinach or kale to boost the nutritional value of your smoothie. Leafy greens are low in oxalates and high in magnesium, which may help prevent the formation of certain types of kidney stones.

- **Protein:** Include a source of lean protein in your smoothie, such as Greek yogurt, tofu, or a plant-based protein powder. Protein helps keep you feeling full and satisfied while supporting muscle health.

- **Healthy Fats:** Add a tablespoon of nut butter, avocado, or chia seeds to your smoothie to incorporate healthy fats. These ingredients provide satiety and promote nutrient absorption.

CHAPTER 5: LUNCHES AND DINNERS

Lean Protein Main Courses

❖ Poultry, Fish, and Lean Meat Recipes

Incorporating poultry, fish, and lean meats into your diet with kidney stone prevention in mind can be both flavorful and beneficial for overall health. Here are some delicious and kidney stone-friendly recipes:

- **Grilled Lemon Herb Chicken:** Marinate boneless, skinless chicken breasts in a mixture of lemon juice, olive oil, garlic, and herbs such as thyme, rosemary, and oregano. Grill until cooked through and serve with a side of steamed green beans and quinoa for a balanced meal low in oxalates and rich in lean protein.

- **Baked Salmon with Dill Sauce:** Season salmon fillets with salt, pepper, and a squeeze of lemon juice. Bake in the oven until flaky. Meanwhile, prepare a dill sauce using Greek yogurt, chopped fresh dill, garlic, and lemon zest. Serve the salmon with the dill sauce alongside roasted asparagus and brown rice for a nutritious and kidney stone-friendly dinner.

- **Turkey and Vegetable Stir-Fry:** Sauté lean ground turkey with a variety of colorful vegetables such as bell peppers, broccoli, carrots, and snap peas in a wok or skillet. Season with ginger, garlic, and low-sodium soy sauce. Serve over cooked brown rice or cauliflower rice for a satisfying and low-oxalate meal.

- **Beef and Vegetable Kabobs:** Thread lean beef cubes onto skewers with cherry tomatoes, onions, and mushrooms. Brush with a marinade made from olive oil, balsamic vinegar, garlic, and herbs. Grill until the beef is cooked to your liking and serve with a side of grilled zucchini and couscous for a kidney stone-friendly barbecue option.

- **Tuna Salad Lettuce Wraps:** Mix canned tuna with Greek yogurt, diced celery, red onion, and lemon juice. Season with salt, pepper, and dill. Spoon the tuna salad into large lettuce leaves and wrap to make lettuce wraps. Serve with a side of sliced cucumber and carrot sticks for a light and refreshing meal that's low in oxalates and high in protein.

Plant-Based Protein Alternatives

For individuals concerned about kidney stone prevention or management, incorporating plant-based protein alternatives into their diet can offer numerous health benefits while minimizing the risk of oxalate accumulation. Here are some kidney stone-friendly plant-based protein options:

- **Lentils:** Lentils are rich in protein, fiber, and essential nutrients while being low in oxalates. They can be used in soups, stews, salads, or as a meat substitute in dishes like lentil tacos or burgers.

- **Chickpeas:** Chickpeas, also known as garbanzo beans, are versatile legumes that are low in oxalates and high in protein. They can be used to make hummus, added to salads, or roasted for a crunchy snack.

- **Quinoa:** Quinoa is a complete protein source, meaning it contains all nine essential amino acids. It's also low in oxalates and can be used as a base for salads, stir-fries, or breakfast bowls.

- **Tofu and Tempeh:** Tofu and tempeh are soy-based protein options that are low in oxalates and provide a good amount of protein per serving. They can be grilled, baked, or stir-fried and added to a variety of dishes.

- **Edamame:** Edamame, or young soybeans, are a delicious and nutritious snack that is low in oxalates and high in protein. They can also be added to salads, stir-fries, or enjoyed on their own as a tasty appetizer.

Portion Control Strategies

Effective portion control is crucial for kidney stone prevention, as excessive intake of certain foods can increase the risk of stone formation. Here are some strategies for practicing portion control to support kidney health:

- **Use Smaller Plates:** Opt for smaller plates and bowls to help control portion sizes visually. Research suggests that people tend to eat less when they use smaller dishware, as it creates the perception of larger portions.

- **Measure Serving Sizes:** Use measuring cups, spoons, or a kitchen scale to accurately portion out foods, especially those high in oxalates or purines, such as nuts, seeds, and grains. This ensures that you're consuming appropriate serving sizes and helps prevent overeating.

- **Fill Half Your Plate with Vegetables:** Aim to fill at least half of your plate with non-starchy vegetables, such as leafy greens, broccoli, and bell peppers. Vegetables are low in oxalates and calories but high in essential nutrients and fiber, promoting satiety and overall health.

- Practice Mindful Eating: Pay attention to hunger and fullness cues and eat slowly to give your body time to register feelings of fullness. Avoid distractions such as television or electronic devices while eating to focus on the sensory experience of food and prevent overeating.

- **Pre-Portion Snacks:** Divide large packages of snacks into single-serving portions to prevent mindless eating and promote portion control. This can help limit intake of high-oxalate snacks like nuts, which should be consumed in moderation.

Kidney-Friendly Sides

❖ **Low-Oxalate Vegetables**

Incorporating low-oxalate vegetables into your diet is an essential component of kidney stone prevention, as high levels of oxalates can contribute to stone formation. Here are some kidney stone-friendly vegetables to include in your meals:

- **Leafy Greens:** Options such as spinach, kale, and Swiss chard are surprisingly low in oxalates compared to other leafy greens. They are also rich in essential nutrients like vitamins A, C, and K, as well as minerals like calcium and magnesium.

- **Bell Peppers:** Bell peppers are not only vibrant and flavorful but also low in oxalates. They provide a good source of vitamin C and other antioxidants, which can help reduce inflammation and support overall kidney health.

- **Zucchini:** Zucchini is a versatile and low-oxalate vegetable that can be enjoyed raw in salads, spiralized into noodles, or grilled as a side dish. It is high in water content, making it hydrating and beneficial for kidney function.

- **Cucumber:** Cucumbers are refreshing, hydrating, and low in oxalates, making them an excellent addition to salads, sandwiches, or as a crunchy snack. They are also low in calories and high in water, promoting hydration and urinary tract health.

- **Cauliflower:** Cauliflower is a cruciferous vegetable that is low in oxalates and can be used as a substitute for higher-oxalate foods like potatoes or rice. It can be roasted, mashed, or riced to create a variety of delicious and kidney stone-friendly dishes.

Whole Grains and Legumes

Whole grains and legumes can be valuable components of a kidney stone-friendly diet due to their low oxalate content and high nutritional value. Including these foods in your meals provides essential nutrients and fiber while helping to prevent the formation of kidney stones.

Whole grains like brown rice, quinoa, barley, and oats are excellent sources of complex carbohydrates, fiber, vitamins, and minerals.

They promote digestive health, regulate blood sugar levels, and provide sustained energy throughout the day. Additionally, their low oxalate content makes them suitable choices for individuals concerned about kidney stone formation.

Legumes such as beans, lentils, and peas are rich in plant-based protein, fiber, and various vitamins and minerals. They offer numerous health benefits, including supporting heart health, managing blood sugar levels, and aiding in weight management. Legumes are also low in oxalates, making them ideal for inclusion in a kidney stone-friendly diet.

Flavorful Herb and Spice Pairings

Flavorful herb and spice pairings can enhance the taste of kidney stone-friendly meals while providing a wide array of health benefits. Here are some delicious combinations that add zest to your dishes while supporting kidney health:

- **Basil and Garlic:** This classic duo not only adds depth of flavor but also offers anti-inflammatory properties. Use them to season pasta sauces, salads, or roasted vegetables.

- **Cilantro and Lime:** The fresh, citrusy taste of lime pairs perfectly with the bright, herbaceous flavor of cilantro. Together, they create a refreshing combination ideal for garnishing soups, tacos, or grilled fish.

- **Rosemary and Lemon:** The earthy aroma of rosemary complements the zesty brightness of lemon, adding a burst of flavor to roasted chicken, potatoes, or vegetables.

- **Turmeric and Ginger:** Known for their anti-inflammatory and antioxidant properties, turmeric and ginger create a warm and spicy flavor profile. Use them to season curries, stir-fries, or smoothies for an extra health boost.

- **Thyme and Sage:** These aromatic herbs bring warmth and depth to dishes like roasted meats, stuffing, or bean soups. Their earthy flavors create a comforting and savory taste experience.

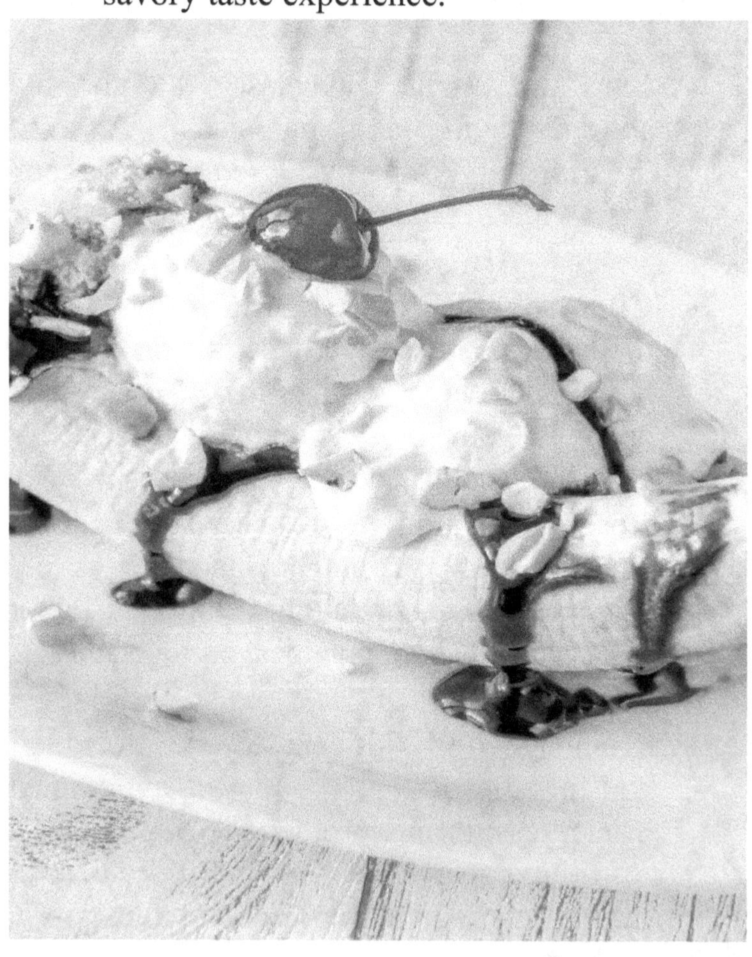

CHAPTER 6: DESSERTS AND TREATS

Fruit-Based Desserts

❖ Berry Sorbets and Fruit Compotes

Berry sorbets and fruit compotes offer delicious ways to satisfy your sweet tooth while supporting kidney stone prevention or management.

These refreshing treats are made from fruits that are low in oxalates and high in water content, making them hydrating and beneficial for kidney health. Here's why berry sorbets and fruit compotes are excellent choices for individuals concerned about kidney stones:

- **Low Oxalate Content**: Berries such as strawberries, blueberries, raspberries, and blackberries are naturally low in oxalates, making them safe options for those prone to kidney stones. By using these fruits as the base for sorbets and compotes, you can enjoy a sweet treat without worrying about increasing your oxalate intake.

- **Hydration:** Both sorbets and fruit compotes contain high water content, which helps promote hydration. Adequate hydration is essential for preventing the formation of kidney stones, as it helps dilute urine and prevents minerals from crystallizing and forming stones in the kidneys.

- **Nutrient-Rich:** Berries are rich in vitamins, minerals, and antioxidants, which offer numerous health benefits. They provide essential nutrients such as vitamin C, manganese, and dietary fiber, which support overall health and kidney function.

- **Versatility:** Berry sorbets and fruit compotes are incredibly versatile and can be customized to suit your taste preferences. You can experiment with different combinations of berries and add natural sweeteners like honey or maple syrup for extra flavor.

- **Enjoyment:** Sorbets and compotes offer a guilt-free way to indulge in something sweet while adhering to a kidney stone-friendly diet. They provide a refreshing and satisfying treat that can be enjoyed on its own or paired with other kidney-friendly desserts like yogurt or angel food cake.

Low-Oxalate Baking Tips

For individuals concerned about kidney stone prevention or management, baking with low-oxalate ingredients can help reduce oxalate intake while still enjoying delicious homemade treats. Here are some tips for baking with low-oxalate ingredients:

- **Choose Low-Oxalate Flours:** Opt for flours that are naturally low in oxalates, such as white flour, oat flour, rice flour, or coconut flour. These alternatives can be used as substitutes for higher-oxalate flours like almond flour or whole wheat flour in recipes for cakes, cookies, muffins, and bread.

- **Incorporate Low-Oxalate Fruits:** Use low-oxalate fruits like apples, pears, bananas, or berries as natural sweeteners and flavor enhancers in baked goods. These fruits can be added to muffins, bread, or cakes for added moisture and sweetness without increasing oxalate levels.

- **Substitute Dairy Wisely:** While dairy products like milk, yogurt, and cheese are generally low in oxalates, some individuals may need to limit their intake due to other dietary restrictions or health concerns. Consider using lactose-free or plant-based alternatives like almond milk, coconut yogurt, or tofu-based cream cheese in your baking recipes.

- **Limit High-Oxalate Add-Ins:** Be cautious with high-oxalate ingredients like nuts, seeds, chocolate, and certain spices (e.g., cinnamon, nutmeg) when baking. Instead, choose low-oxalate alternatives or use them sparingly to minimize oxalate intake.

- **Balance Your Diet:** While baking with low-oxalate ingredients is beneficial for kidney stone prevention, it's essential to maintain a balanced diet that includes a variety of nutrient-dense foods. Incorporate plenty of fruits, vegetables, lean proteins, and whole grains into your meals to support overall kidney health.

Sweet Snack Ideas

When it comes to satisfying your sweet tooth while prioritizing kidney stone prevention or management, there are plenty of delicious options that won't increase your risk of stone formation. Here are some sweet snack ideas that are low in oxalates and high in nutrients:

- **Fruit Salad:** Create a colorful fruit salad using low-oxalate fruits such as apples, pears, berries, and melons. Sprinkle with a squeeze of lemon juice or a drizzle of honey for extra flavor. This refreshing snack is hydrating and packed with vitamins, minerals, and antioxidants.

- **Greek Yogurt with Honey and Berries:** Enjoy a serving of plain Greek yogurt topped with fresh berries and a drizzle of honey. Greek yogurt is a rich source of protein and calcium, while berries provide natural sweetness and antioxidants. This creamy and satisfying snack is perfect for satisfying cravings without compromising kidney health.

- **Rice Cake with Almond Butter and Banana Slices:** Spread a rice cake with almond butter and top with thinly sliced banana for a satisfying and low-oxalate snack. Almond butter provides healthy fats and protein, while bananas offer natural sweetness and potassium. This snack is quick, easy, and perfect for on-the-go.

- **Cottage Cheese with Pineapple:** Enjoy a serving of low-fat cottage cheese paired with chunks of fresh pineapple. Cottage cheese is a good source of protein and calcium, while pineapple provides natural sweetness and bromelain, an enzyme that may help support digestion and reduce inflammation.

- **Baked Apples with Cinnamon:** Core an apple and sprinkle with cinnamon before baking until tender. This simple yet satisfying snack is naturally sweet and comforting, making it an excellent choice for a kidney stone-friendly treat.

Moderation and Indulgence

- **Dessert Portion Control**

Dessert portion control is essential for kidney stone prevention or management, as certain sweet treats can contribute to the formation of kidney stones if consumed in excess. Here are some tips for practicing portion control while still enjoying dessert:

- **Use Smaller Servings:** Opt for smaller servings of desserts to help control portion sizes. Instead of indulging in a large slice of cake or a giant scoop of ice cream, aim for a smaller portion that satisfies your sweet tooth without overdoing it.

- **Share Desserts:** If dining out or enjoying dessert at home, consider sharing a dessert with a friend or family member. Splitting a dessert allows you to enjoy a taste of something sweet without consuming a full portion.

- **Choose Mini Versions:** Look for mini or individual-sized desserts when available. Mini cupcakes, petit fours, or single-serving ice cream cups are great options that provide built-in portion control.

- **Practice Mindful Eating:** Pay attention to hunger and fullness cues while enjoying dessert. Eat slowly, savoring each bite, and stop when you feel satisfied rather than overly full. This mindful approach to eating can help prevent overindulgence.

- **Opt for Lower-Calorie Options:** Choose desserts that are lower in calories and sugar to help keep portions in check. Fresh fruit, frozen yogurt, or angel food cake are lighter alternatives that still satisfy a sweet craving without adding excess calories or sugar.

- **Plan Ahead:** Plan dessert into your overall meal plan and budget your calories accordingly. By planning ahead, you can enjoy dessert guilt-free while staying within your daily calorie goals.

- **Treat Dessert as an Occasional Indulgence:** Reserve dessert for special occasions or as an occasional treat rather than a daily indulgence. This approach allows you to enjoy dessert in moderation while prioritizing overall kidney health.

Occasional Treats

Occasional treats can be enjoyed in moderation as part of a kidney stone-friendly diet, allowing individuals to satisfy cravings while still prioritizing kidney health. Here are some tips for incorporating occasional treats into your diet:

- **Plan Ahead:** Schedule occasional treats into your meal plan to ensure they fit within your overall dietary goals. By planning ahead, you can enjoy treats without feeling guilty or compromising your kidney stone prevention efforts.

- **Choose Wisely:** When indulging in occasional treats, opt for options that are lower in oxalates, sugar, and unhealthy fats. For example, choose dark chocolate instead of milk chocolate, or opt for sorbet instead of ice cream. This allows you to enjoy a sweet treat while minimizing the risk of kidney stone formation.

- **Practice Portion Control:** Enjoy treats in moderation and practice portion control to prevent overindulgence. Instead of eating an entire slice of cake or a full bag of chips, have a small serving and savor each bite.

- **Balance with Nutrient-Dense Foods:** Offset occasional treats by incorporating nutrient-dense foods into your diet. Focus on eating plenty of fruits, vegetables, whole grains, and lean proteins to ensure you're meeting your nutritional needs while still enjoying treats in moderation.

- **Stay Hydrated:** Drink plenty of water before and after enjoying occasional treats to help flush out any excess minerals and prevent the formation of kidney stones. Staying hydrated is essential for kidney health and can help mitigate the impact of occasional indulgences.

- **Mindful Eating:** Practice mindful eating when enjoying occasional treats by paying attention to hunger and fullness cues, eating slowly, and savoring each bite. This allows you to fully enjoy the treat and prevents mindless overeating.

Smart Swaps for Sweet Cravings

When experiencing sweet cravings while prioritizing kidney stone prevention or management, making smart swaps can satisfy your taste buds while supporting kidney health. Here are some tips for swapping high-oxalate or sugary sweets with healthier alternatives:

- **Fresh Fruit Instead of Candy:** Instead of reaching for candy or other sugary snacks, opt for fresh fruit to satisfy your sweet cravings. Fruits like berries, grapes, melons, and oranges are naturally sweet and low in oxalates, making them excellent choices for kidney stone-friendly snacks.

- **Dark Chocolate Instead of Milk Chocolate:** Dark chocolate contains less sugar and is lower in oxalates compared to milk chocolate. Choose dark chocolate with a higher cocoa content (70% or higher) for a rich, indulgent treat that provides antioxidants and may even offer health benefits.

- **Frozen Yogurt Instead of Ice Cream:** Swap traditional ice cream for frozen yogurt or Greek yogurt-based frozen treats. Frozen yogurt is lower in fat and sugar than ice cream and provides probiotics that support gut health. Look for varieties without added sugars or artificial sweeteners for a healthier option.

- **Homemade Baked Goods with Low-Oxalate Flours:** Bake your own sweet treats using low-oxalate flours like white flour, oat flour, or rice flour. Experiment with recipes for cookies, muffins, and cakes using these alternative flours to reduce oxalate intake while still satisfying your sweet tooth.

- **Trail Mix with Nuts and Dried Fruit:** Create your own trail mix using a combination of nuts and dried fruits. Choose nuts like almonds, cashews, and pistachios, which are lower in oxalates, and pair them with dried fruits like apricots, cherries, or raisins for a sweet and satisfying snack.

- **Fruit Smoothies Instead of Sugary Drinks:** Blend up a fruit smoothie using low-oxalate fruits, yogurt, and a splash of almond milk or coconut water for sweetness. Avoid adding sugary syrups or sweetened juices and opt for natural sweeteners like honey or maple syrup if needed.

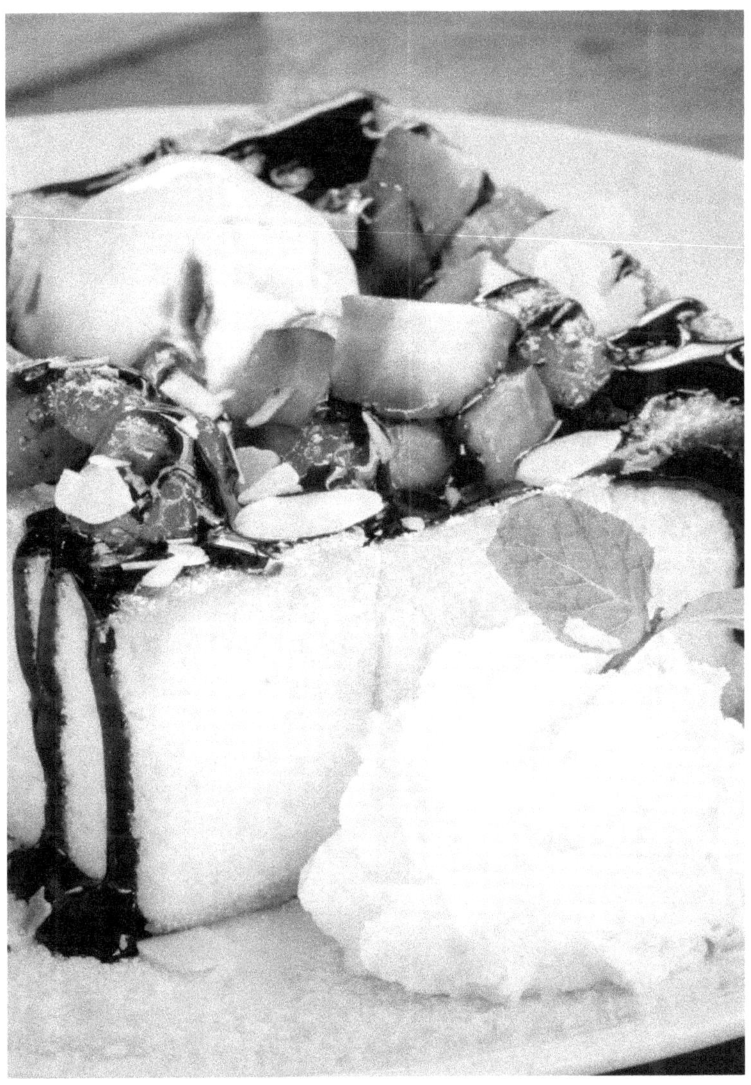

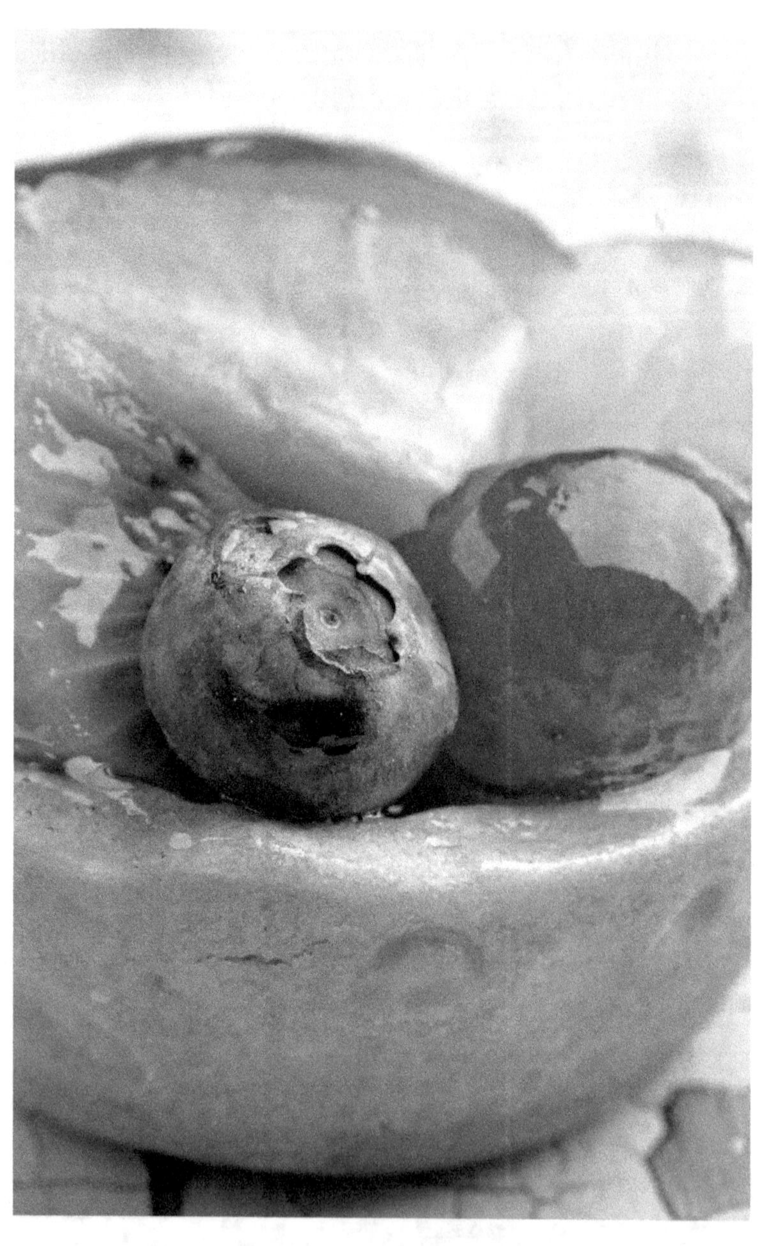

CHAPTER 7: MEAL PLANNING AND SAMPLE MENUS

Weekly Meal Planning Guide

❖ Balancing Nutrients

Balancing nutrients is crucial for kidney stone prevention or management, as certain dietary factors can either increase or decrease the risk of stone formation. Here's how to balance nutrients effectively to support kidney health:

- **Hydration:** Adequate hydration is essential for kidney stone prevention, as it helps dilute urine and prevent minerals from crystallizing and forming stones in the kidneys. Aim to drink at least 8-10 cups of water per day, and increase your fluid intake during hot weather or when engaging in physical activity.

- **Calcium:** Contrary to popular belief, consuming adequate amounts of calcium is important for kidney stone prevention. Calcium binds with oxalates in the intestines, reducing their absorption and excretion in the urine. Include calcium-rich foods such as low-fat dairy products, leafy greens, tofu, and fortified foods in your diet.

- **Magnesium:** Magnesium plays a role in preventing the formation of certain types of kidney stones by inhibiting the crystallization of calcium oxalate in the urine. Include magnesium-rich foods like nuts, seeds, whole grains, and leafy greens in your diet.

- **Potassium:** Potassium helps regulate fluid balance and reduce the risk of kidney stone formation by increasing urinary citrate levels, which inhibit the formation of calcium stones. Include potassium-rich foods such as bananas, oranges, potatoes, spinach, and avocados in your diet.

- **Fiber:** Dietary fiber helps prevent constipation and promotes regular bowel movements, which can reduce the absorption of oxalates in the gut. Include fiber-rich foods like fruits, vegetables, whole grains, legumes, and nuts in your diet.

- **Limit Sodium:** Excess sodium can increase the risk of kidney stone formation by increasing urinary calcium excretion. Limit your intake of processed foods, canned soups, salty snacks, and fast food, and opt for fresh or minimally processed foods instead.
- **Limit Oxalate-Rich Foods:** While oxalates are found naturally in many plant foods, consuming them in excessive amounts can increase the risk of calcium oxalate kidney stones.

- Limit your intake of high-oxalate foods like spinach, rhubarb, beets, nuts, seeds, and chocolate, and choose lower-oxalate alternatives whenever possible.

- **Moderate Protein Intake:** While protein is an essential nutrient, consuming excessive amounts of animal protein can increase the risk of kidney stones, particularly uric acid stones. Aim for moderate amounts of lean protein sources like poultry, fish, tofu, legumes, and nuts.

Creating Varied Menus

Creating varied menus for kidney stone prevention or management is essential to ensure you're getting a wide range of nutrients while minimizing the risk of stone formation. Here's how to create diverse and kidney stone-friendly menus:

- **Incorporate a Variety of Fruits and Vegetables:** Aim to include a colorful array of fruits and vegetables in your menus to provide essential vitamins, minerals, and antioxidants. Choose low-oxalate options such as apples, berries, melons, cucumbers, bell peppers, and leafy greens. Rotate your selection regularly to ensure you're getting a diverse range of nutrients.

- **Include Lean Proteins:** Incorporate lean sources of protein into your menus to support muscle health and satiety. Choose options like skinless poultry, fish, tofu, legumes, and low-fat dairy products. Experiment with different cooking methods and flavorings to keep meals interesting and flavorful.

- **Opt for Whole Grains:** Choose whole grains like brown rice, quinoa, barley, oats, and whole wheat bread or pasta to provide fiber, vitamins, and minerals. These options are lower in oxalates compared to refined grains and offer a variety of textures and flavors to keep your menus interesting.

- **Add Healthy Fats:** Include sources of healthy fats in your menus such as nuts, seeds, avocados, and olive oil. These fats provide essential fatty acids and fat-soluble vitamins while adding richness and flavor to your meals. Use them in moderation to balance your overall diet.

- **Experiment with Herbs and Spices:** Use herbs, spices, and aromatics to add depth and complexity to your menus without relying on high-oxalate ingredients like salt or processed sauces. Experiment with fresh herbs like basil, cilantro, mint, and rosemary, as well as spices like turmeric, ginger, cumin, and paprika.

- **Plan Balanced Meals:** Ensure each meal contains a balance of carbohydrates, protein, and healthy fats, along with plenty of fruits and vegetables. Aim for variety within each meal by including different food groups, textures, and flavors.

- **Try New Recipes:** Keep your menus exciting and varied by trying new recipes regularly. Explore different cuisines, cooking techniques, and ingredients to keep your taste buds engaged and your meals enjoyable.

- **Stay Hydrated:** Remember to drink plenty of water throughout the day to support kidney health and prevent dehydration, which can increase the risk of kidney stone formation. Consider incorporating hydrating foods like soups, smoothies, and watery fruits and vegetables into your menus.

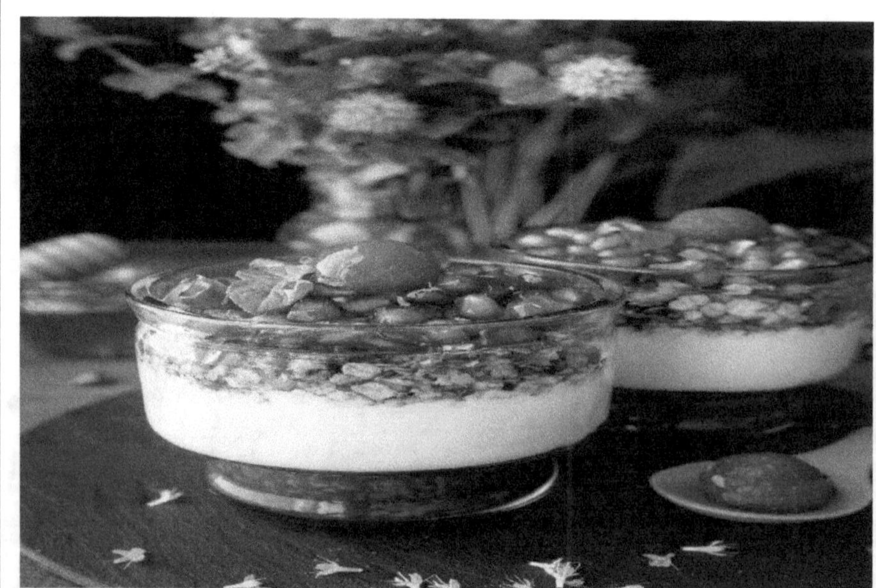

Shopping List Essentials

When creating a shopping list for kidney stone prevention or management, it's essential to include a variety of nutrient-dense foods that support kidney health while minimizing the risk of stone formation. Here are some shopping list essentials for a kidney stone-friendly diet:

- **Low-Oxalate Fruits:** Stock up on low-oxalate fruits such as apples, berries (strawberries, blueberries, raspberries), melons (watermelon, cantaloupe, honeydew), bananas, and citrus fruits (oranges, lemons, limes). These fruits are hydrating and provide essential vitamins, minerals, and antioxidants.

- **Low-Oxalate Vegetables:** Choose a variety of low-oxalate vegetables like leafy greens (spinach, kale, Swiss chard), bell peppers, cucumbers, carrots, zucchini, and cauliflower. These vegetables are rich in fiber, vitamins, and minerals while being gentle on the kidneys.

- **Lean Proteins:** Include lean sources of protein in your shopping list such as skinless poultry (chicken, turkey), fish (salmon, tuna, cod), tofu, tempeh, legumes (beans, lentils), and low-fat dairy products (Greek yogurt, cottage cheese). These protein sources support muscle health and provide essential nutrients without contributing to kidney stone formation.

- **Whole Grains:** Opt for whole grains like brown rice, quinoa, barley, oats, whole wheat bread, and whole grain pasta. These grains are lower in oxalates compared to refined grains and provide fiber, vitamins, and minerals to support overall health.

- **Healthy Fats:** Choose sources of healthy fats such as nuts (almonds, walnuts, pistachios), seeds (chia seeds, flaxseeds, pumpkin seeds), avocados, and olive oil. These fats provide essential fatty acids and fat-soluble vitamins while adding richness and flavor to your meals.

- **Hydration:** Don't forget to include water on your shopping list to stay hydrated throughout the day. Consider also purchasing herbal teas, coconut water, or sparkling water for variety.

- **Herbs and Spices:** Stock up on a variety of herbs, spices, and aromatics to add flavor to your meals without relying on high-oxalate ingredients. Experiment with fresh herbs like basil, cilantro, mint, and rosemary, as well as spices like turmeric, ginger, cumin, and paprika.

Sample meal plan

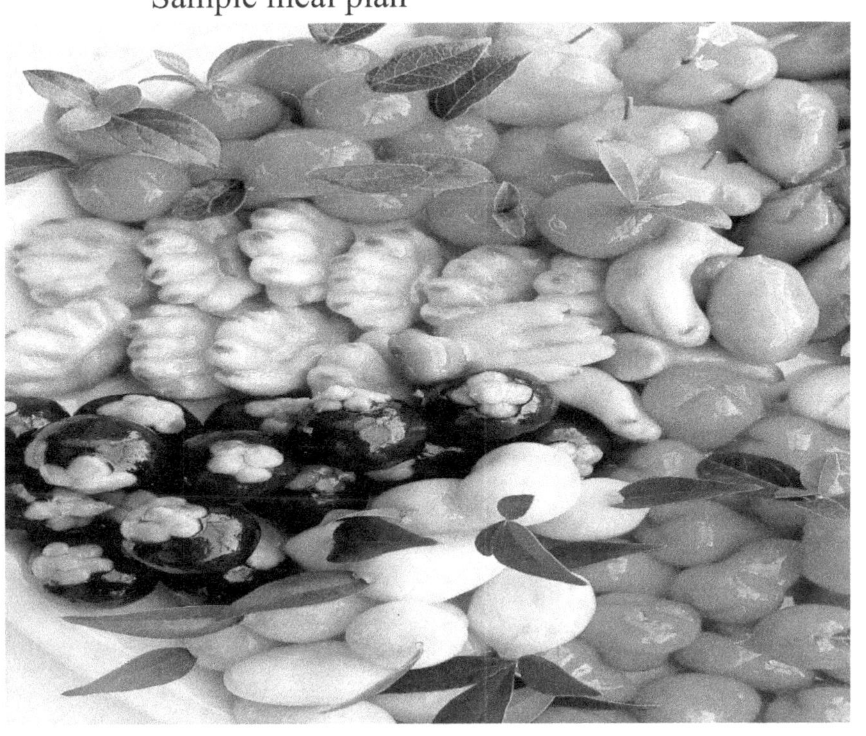

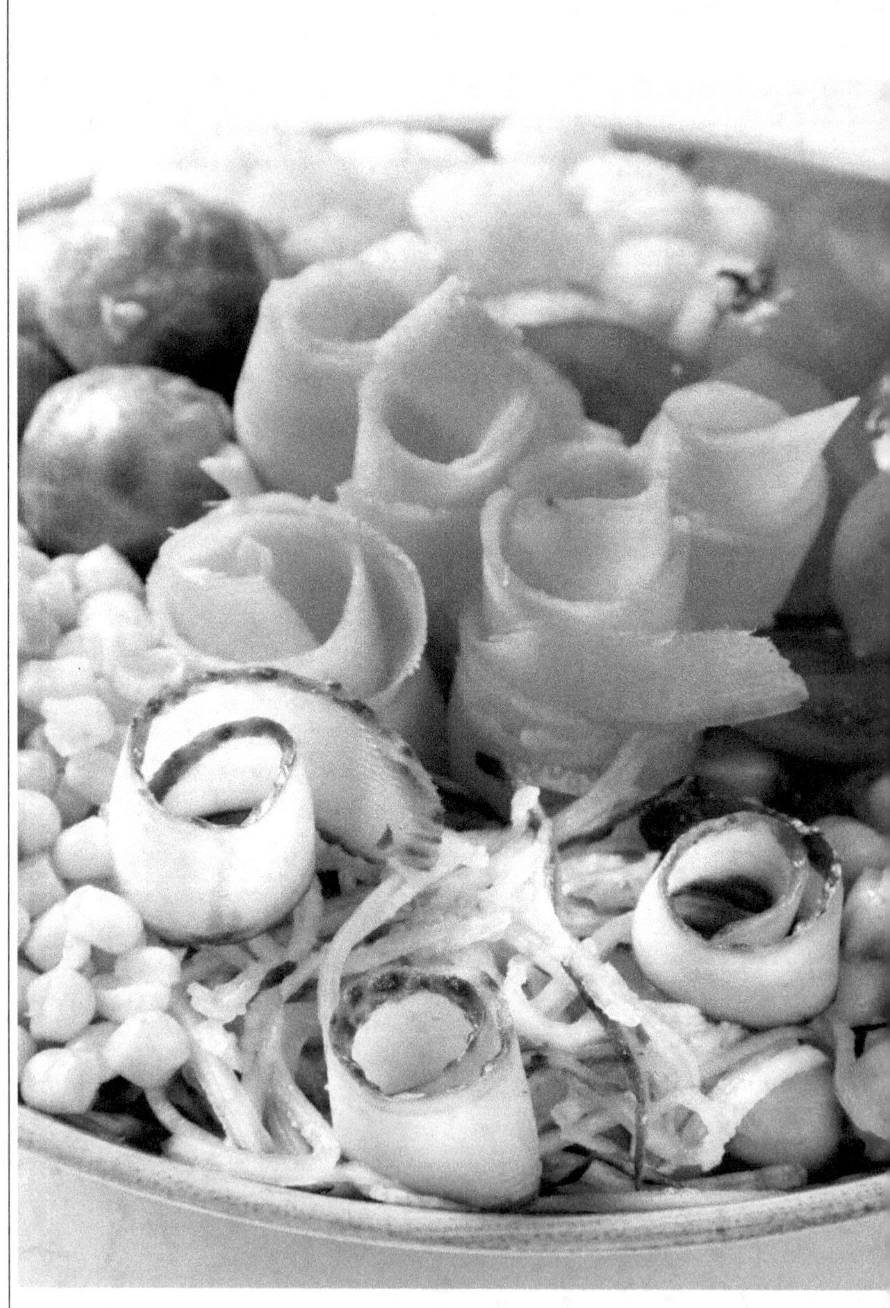

CHAPTER 8: 7-DAY MEAL PLAN FOR KIDNEY STONE

Day 1:
Breakfast: Blueberry Oatmeal
Ingredients:
- ❖ 1/2 cup rolled oats
- ❖ 1 cup almond milk
- ❖ 1/4 cup blueberries
- ❖ 1 tablespoon honey
- ❖ 1 tablespoon chopped almonds

Instructions:
1. In a small saucepan, bring almond milk to a boil.
2. Stir in rolled oats and reduce heat to low. Cook for 5-7 minutes, stirring occasionally, until oats are tender.
3. Remove from heat and stir in blueberries and honey.
4. Serve hot, garnished with chopped almonds.
- ❖ Prep Time: 10 minutes

Lunch: Quinoa and Vegetable Salad
Ingredients:
- ❖ 1/2 cup quinoa, rinsed
- ❖ 1 cup water
- ❖ 1/2 cup diced cucumber

* ❖ 1/2 cup cherry tomatoes, halved
* ❖ 1/4 cup chopped bell pepper
* ❖ 2 tablespoons chopped parsley
* ❖ 1 tablespoon olive oil
* ❖ 1 tablespoon lemon juice
* ❖ Salt and pepper to taste

Instructions:

1. In a saucepan, combine quinoa and water. Bring to a boil, then reduce heat to low, cover, and simmer for 15 minutes.
2. Remove from heat and let stand for 5 minutes, then fluff with a fork and let cool.
3. In a large bowl, combine cooked quinoa, cucumber, tomatoes, bell pepper, and parsley.
4. In a small bowl, whisk together olive oil, lemon juice, salt, and pepper. Pour over the quinoa mixture and toss to combine.
5. Serve chilled or at room temperature.

* ❖ Prep Time: 20 minutes

Dinner: Grilled Lemon Herb Chicken with Steamed Asparagus

Ingredients:

* ❖ 4 boneless, skinless chicken breasts
* ❖ 2 tablespoons olive oil
* ❖ 2 tablespoons lemon juice
* ❖ 2 cloves garlic, minced

- ❖ 1 teaspoon dried thyme
- ❖ 1 teaspoon dried rosemary
- ❖ Salt and pepper to taste
- ❖ 1 bunch asparagus, trimmed

Instructions:

1. In a bowl, whisk together olive oil, lemon juice, garlic, thyme, rosemary, salt, and pepper.
2. Place chicken breasts in a resealable plastic bag and pour marinade over them. Seal the bag and refrigerate for at least 30 minutes.
3. Preheat grill to medium-high heat. Remove chicken from marinade and discard excess marinade.
4. Grill chicken for 6-8 minutes per side, or until cooked through and no longer pink in the center.
5. While chicken is grilling, steam asparagus until tender-crisp, about 4-5 minutes.
6. Serve grilled chicken with steamed asparagus.

- ❖ Prep Time: 40 minutes

Day 2:
Breakfast: Greek Yogurt Parfait
Ingredients:

- ❖ 1 cup plain Greek yogurt
- ❖ 1/4 cup granola
- ❖ 1/4 cup mixed berries (such as strawberries, raspberries, and blueberries)
- ❖ 1 tablespoon honey

Instructions:

1. In a glass or bowl, layer Greek yogurt, granola, and mixed berries.
2. Drizzle with honey.
3. Serve immediately.
- ❖ Prep Time: 5 minutes

Lunch: Lentil Soup
Ingredients:

- ❖ 1 cup dried lentils, rinsed
- ❖ 4 cups vegetable broth
- ❖ 1 onion, diced
- ❖ 2 carrots, diced
- ❖ 2 celery stalks, diced
- ❖ 2 cloves garlic, minced
- ❖ 1 teaspoon cumin
- ❖ 1 teaspoon paprika
- ❖ Salt and pepper to taste
- ❖ 2 tablespoons chopped parsley

Instructions:

1. In a large pot, combine lentils, vegetable broth, onion, carrots, celery, garlic, cumin, paprika, salt, and pepper.
2. Bring to a boil, then reduce heat to low and simmer for 25-30 minutes, or until lentils and vegetables are tender.
3. Stir in chopped parsley before serving.
❖ Prep Time: 10 minutes

Dinner: Baked Salmon with Roasted Vegetables
Ingredients:
❖ 4 salmon fillets
❖ 2 tablespoons olive oil
❖ 1 tablespoon lemon juice
❖ 2 cloves garlic, minced
❖ 1 teaspoon dried dill
❖ Salt and pepper to taste
❖ 2 cups mixed vegetables (such as bell peppers, zucchini, and cherry tomatoes), chopped

Instructions:

1. Preheat oven to 400°F (200°C).
2. In a small bowl, whisk together olive oil, lemon juice, garlic, dill, salt, and pepper.
3. Place salmon fillets on a baking sheet lined with parchment paper. Brush salmon with the olive oil mixture.

4. Toss mixed vegetables with the remaining olive oil mixture and spread them around the salmon on the baking sheet.
5. Bake for 12-15 minutes, or until salmon is cooked through and vegetables are tender.
6. Serve baked salmon with roasted vegetables.
- ❖ Prep Time: 25 minutes

Day 3:
Breakfast: Spinach and Feta Omelette
Ingredients:
- ❖ 2 eggs
- ❖ 1 tablespoon water
- ❖ 1 cup fresh spinach leaves
- ❖ 2 tablespoons crumbled feta cheese
- ❖ Salt and pepper to taste
- ❖ 1 teaspoon olive oil

Instructions:
1. In a small bowl, whisk together eggs and water until frothy.
2. Heat olive oil in a non-stick skillet over medium heat. Add spinach and cook until wilted.
3. Pour the egg mixture over the spinach in the skillet. Cook for 2-3 minutes, lifting the edges with a spatula to let the uncooked eggs flow underneath.

4. Sprinkle feta cheese over half of the omelette. Fold the other half over the filling and cook for another 1-2 minutes, or until eggs are set.
5. Slide the omelette onto a plate and season with salt and pepper to taste.
❖ Prep Time: 10 minutes

Lunch: Chickpea Salad
Ingredients:
- ❖ 1 can (15 oz) chickpeas, drained and rinsed
- ❖ 1 cucumber, diced
- ❖ 1 bell pepper, diced
- ❖ 1/4 cup diced red onion
- ❖ 2 tablespoons chopped parsley
- ❖ 2 tablespoons lemon juice
- ❖ 1 tablespoon olive oil
- ❖ Salt and pepper to taste

Instructions:
1. In a large bowl, combine chickpeas, cucumber, bell pepper, red onion, and parsley.
2. In a small bowl, whisk together lemon juice, olive oil, salt, and pepper.
3. Pour dressing over the chickpea mixture and toss to combine.
4. Serve chilled or at room temperature.

Prep Time: 15 minutes

Dinner: Turkey and Vegetable Stir-Fry
Ingredients:
- ❖ 1 tablespoon olive oil
- ❖ 1 lb turkey breast, sliced into thin strips
- ❖ 2 cups mixed vegetables (such as broccoli, bell peppers, and snap peas), sliced
- ❖ 2 cloves garlic, minced
- ❖ 1 tablespoon grated ginger
- ❖ 2 tablespoons low-sodium soy sauce
- ❖ 1 tablespoon honey
- ❖ Cooked brown rice for serving

Instructions:
1. Heat olive oil in a large skillet or wok over medium-high heat.
2. Add turkey strips and cook for 3-4 minutes, or until browned and cooked through. Remove turkey from skillet and set aside.
3. In the same skillet, add mixed vegetables, garlic, and ginger. Stir-fry for 2-3 minutes, or until vegetables are tender-crisp.
4. Return cooked turkey to the skillet. Add soy sauce and honey, stirring to coat everything evenly.
5. Cook for another 1-2 minutes, or until heated through.

6. Serve turkey and vegetable stir-fry over cooked brown rice.
* Prep Time: 25 minutes

Day 4:

Breakfast: Avocado Toast with Poached Egg

Ingredients:
* 1 slice whole grain bread, toasted
* 1/2 ripe avocado, mashed
* 1 poached egg
* Salt and pepper to taste
* Optional toppings: red pepper flakes, sliced cherry tomatoes, chopped cilantro

Instructions:
1. Spread mashed avocado evenly onto toasted bread.
2. Top with a poached egg.
3. Season with salt and pepper to taste.
4. Garnish with optional toppings if desired.
5. Serve immediately.
* Prep Time: 15 minutes

Lunch: Spinach and Strawberry Salad

Ingredients:
* 2 cups baby spinach leaves
* 1/2 cup sliced strawberries
* 1/4 cup crumbled goat cheese
* 2 tablespoons balsamic vinaigrette dressing

Instructions:

1. In a large bowl, combine baby spinach, sliced strawberries, and crumbled goat cheese.
2. Drizzle with balsamic vinaigrette dressing and toss to coat.
3. Serve immediately.
❖ Prep Time: 10 minutes

Dinner: Lemon Herb Baked Cod with Steamed Green Beans

Ingredients:

❖ 4 cod fillets
❖ 2 tablespoons olive oil
❖ 2 tablespoons lemon juice
❖ 2 cloves garlic, minced
❖ 1 teaspoon dried thyme
❖ 1 teaspoon dried parsley
❖ Salt and pepper to taste
❖ 1 lb green beans, trimmed

Instructions:

1. Preheat oven to 400°F (200°C).
2. In a small bowl, whisk together olive oil, lemon juice, garlic, thyme, parsley, salt, and pepper.
3. Place cod fillets on a baking sheet lined with parchment paper. Brush cod with the olive oil mixture.

4. Bake for 12-15 minutes, or until cod is opaque and flakes easily with a fork.
5. While cod is baking, steam green beans until tender-crisp, about 4-5 minutes.
6. Serve baked cod with steamed green beans.
❖ Prep Time: 25 minutes

Day 5:
Breakfast: Berry Smoothie Bowl
Ingredients:
❖ 1/2 cup frozen mixed berries
❖ 1/2 banana
❖ 1/2 cup plain Greek yogurt
❖ 1/4 cup almond milk
❖ 1 tablespoon honey
❖ Toppings: granola, sliced bananas, shredded coconut, chia seeds

Instructions:
1. In a blender, combine frozen berries, banana, Greek yogurt, almond milk, and honey. Blend until smooth.
2. Pour smoothie into a bowl.
3. Top with granola, sliced bananas, shredded coconut, and chia seeds.
4. Serve immediately.
❖ Prep Time: 5 minutes

Lunch: Mediterranean Chickpea Salad
Ingredients:
- ❖ 1 can (15 oz) chickpeas, drained and rinsed
- ❖ 1 cucumber, diced
- ❖ 1 bell pepper, diced
- ❖ 1/4 cup diced red onion
- ❖ 1/4 cup chopped Kalamata olives
- ❖ 2 tablespoons chopped parsley
- ❖ 2 tablespoons lemon juice
- ❖ 1 tablespoon olive oil
- ❖ Salt and pepper to taste

Instructions:
1. In a large bowl, combine chickpeas, cucumber, bell pepper, red onion, olives, and parsley.
2. In a small bowl, whisk together lemon juice, olive oil, salt, and pepper.
3. Pour dressing over the chickpea mixture and toss to combine.
4. Serve chilled or at room temperature.
- ❖ Prep Time: 15 minutes

Dinner: Vegetable Stir-Fried Rice
Ingredients:
- ❖ 2 cups cooked brown rice, chilled
- ❖ 2 tablespoons olive oil
- ❖ 2 cloves garlic, minced
- ❖ 1 teaspoon grated ginger

- ❖ 1 cup mixed vegetables (such as carrots, peas, and corn)
- ❖ 2 eggs, lightly beaten
- ❖ 2 tablespoons low-sodium soy sauce
- ❖ 1 tablespoon rice vinegar
- ❖ Salt and pepper to taste
- ❖ 2 green onions, sliced

Instructions:

1. Heat olive oil in a large skillet or wok over medium-high heat.
2. Add garlic and ginger, and stir-fry for 1 minute.
3. Add mixed vegetables and stir-fry for 3-4 minutes, or until tender.
4. Push vegetables to one side of the skillet and pour beaten eggs into the empty space. Scramble eggs until cooked through.
5. Add cooked brown rice to the skillet, breaking up any clumps with a spatula.
6. Stir in soy sauce, rice vinegar, salt, and pepper. Cook for another 2-3 minutes, or until heated through.
7. Garnish with sliced green onions before serving.

- ❖ Prep Time: 30 minutes

Day 6:
Breakfast: Spinach and Mushroom Frittata
Ingredients:

* 6 eggs
* 1/4 cup milk
* 1 cup fresh spinach leaves
* 1 cup sliced mushrooms
* 1/4 cup shredded mozzarella cheese
* Salt and pepper to taste
* 1 teaspoon olive oil

Instructions:

1. Preheat oven to 350°F (175°C).
2. In a bowl, whisk together eggs and milk until well combined. Season with salt and pepper.
3. Heat olive oil in an oven-safe skillet over medium heat. Add spinach and mushrooms, and cook until spinach is wilted and mushrooms are tender.
4. Pour egg mixture over the spinach and mushrooms in the skillet. Sprinkle shredded mozzarella cheese on top.
5. Transfer skillet to the preheated oven and bake for 15-20 minutes, or until eggs are set.
6. Remove from oven and let cool slightly before slicing and serving.

* Prep Time: 20 minutes

Lunch: Caprese Salad
Ingredients:

- ❖ 2 large tomatoes, sliced
- ❖ 1 ball fresh mozzarella cheese, sliced
- ❖ 1/4 cup fresh basil leaves
- ❖ 2 tablespoons balsamic glaze
- ❖ Salt and pepper to taste

Instructions:

1. Arrange tomato and mozzarella slices alternately on a serving plate.
2. Tuck fresh basil leaves between the tomato and mozzarella slices.
3. Drizzle with balsamic glaze and season with salt and pepper to taste.
4. Serve immediately.
- ❖ Prep Time: 10 minutes

Dinner: Lemon Herb Grilled Chicken with Roasted Vegetables
Ingredients:

- ❖ 4 boneless, skinless chicken breasts
- ❖ 2 tablespoons olive oil
- ❖ 2 tablespoons lemon juice
- ❖ 2 cloves garlic, minced
- ❖ 1 teaspoon dried thyme
- ❖ 1 teaspoon dried oregano
- ❖ Salt and pepper to taste

❖ 2 cups mixed vegetables (such as carrots, bell peppers, and onions), chopped

Instructions:

1. In a bowl, whisk together olive oil, lemon juice, garlic, thyme, oregano, salt, and pepper.
2. Place chicken breasts in a resealable plastic bag and pour marinade over them. Seal the bag and refrigerate for at least 30 minutes.
3. Preheat grill to medium-high heat. Remove chicken from marinade and discard excess marinade.
4. Grill chicken for 6-8 minutes per side, or until cooked through and no longer pink in the center.
5. While chicken is grilling, toss mixed vegetables with a drizzle of olive oil, salt, and pepper. Spread them on a baking sheet and roast in the oven at 400°F (200°C) for 15-20 minutes, or until tender.
6. Serve grilled chicken with roasted vegetables.

❖ Prep Time: 40 minutes

Day 7:
Breakfast: Veggie Breakfast Burrito
Ingredients:

- ❖ 2 large eggs
- ❖ 1/4 cup diced bell peppers
- ❖ 1/4 cup diced onions
- ❖ 1/4 cup diced tomatoes
- ❖ 2 tablespoons shredded cheddar cheese
- ❖ 2 whole wheat tortillas
- ❖ Salt and pepper to taste
- ❖ Optional toppings: salsa, avocado slices, Greek yogurt

Instructions:

1. In a small bowl, whisk together eggs, salt, and pepper.
2. Heat a non-stick skillet over medium heat. Add diced bell peppers and onions, and cook for 2-3 minutes until softened.
3. Add diced tomatoes to the skillet and cook for another 1-2 minutes.
4. Pour the whisked eggs into the skillet and scramble until cooked through.
5. Divide scrambled eggs evenly between two whole wheat tortillas. Sprinkle shredded cheddar cheese on top.
6. Roll up the tortillas to form burritos.
7. Serve immediately with optional toppings if desired.

❖ Prep Time: 15 minutes

Lunch: Turkey and Avocado Wrap
Ingredients:
- ❖ 2 whole wheat wraps
- ❖ 4 slices turkey breast
- ❖ 1/2 avocado, sliced
- ❖ 1/4 cup shredded lettuce
- ❖ 1/4 cup diced tomatoes
- ❖ 2 tablespoons hummus

Instructions:
1. Lay whole wheat wraps flat on a clean surface.
2. Spread hummus evenly over each wrap.
3. Place turkey slices, avocado slices, shredded lettuce, and diced tomatoes down the center of each wrap.
4. Roll up the wraps tightly.
5. Slice in half and serve immediately.
- ❖ Prep Time: 10 minutes

Dinner: Lentil and Vegetable Curry
Ingredients:
- ❖ 1 cup dried lentils, rinsed
- ❖ 4 cups vegetable broth
- ❖ 1 onion, diced
- ❖ 2 cloves garlic, minced
- ❖ 1 tablespoon grated ginger

- ❖ 1 tablespoon curry powder
- ❖ 1 teaspoon turmeric
- ❖ 1 can (14 oz) diced tomatoes
- ❖ 2 cups mixed vegetables (such as carrots, cauliflower, and peas)
- ❖ Salt and pepper to taste
- ❖ Cooked brown rice for serving
- ❖ Fresh cilantro for garnish

Instructions:

1. In a large pot, combine lentils, vegetable broth, onion, garlic, ginger, curry powder, turmeric, diced tomatoes, mixed vegetables, salt, and pepper.
2. Bring to a boil, then reduce heat to low and simmer for 20-25 minutes, or until lentils and vegetables are tender.
3. Serve lentil and vegetable curry over cooked brown rice.
4. Garnish with fresh cilantro before serving.

- ❖ Prep Time: 30 minutes

Special Occasion Menus

Special occasions provide an opportunity to enjoy delicious meals while still prioritizing kidney stone prevention or management. Here's how to create special occasion menus that are both celebratory and kidney stone-friendly:

- **Appetizers:** Start the meal with light and flavorful appetizers that won't overload the kidneys. Opt for options like a shrimp cocktail with a tangy cocktail sauce,
- a Greek salad with fresh vegetables and feta cheese, or bruschetta topped with diced tomatoes, basil, and a drizzle of balsamic glaze. These appetizers are refreshing and satisfying without being overly heavy.

- **Main Course:** For the main course, choose protein-rich dishes that are cooked with kidney stone-friendly ingredients. Consider options like grilled salmon with a lemon-dill sauce, herb-roasted chicken breast with roasted vegetables, or a vegetable and tofu stir-fry served over brown rice. These dishes are nutritious, flavorful, and sure to impress your guests.

- **Side Dishes:** Complement the main course with a variety of kidney stone-friendly side dishes. Serve steamed asparagus with a squeeze of lemon, quinoa pilaf with mixed herbs and vegetables, or roasted sweet potatoes with a sprinkle of cinnamon. These side dishes add color and texture to the meal while providing essential nutrients.

- **Desserts:** Indulge your sweet tooth with desserts that are light and satisfying. Opt for options like fresh fruit platters with a yogurt dipping sauce, baked apples stuffed with oats and cinnamon, or a berry sorbet garnished with mint leaves. These desserts provide a sweet ending to the meal without adding unnecessary sugar or calories.

- **Beverages:** Offer a selection of hydrating beverages to accompany the meal. Serve infused water with cucumber and mint, herbal teas with lemon and ginger, or sparkling water with a splash of fruit juice. These beverages are refreshing and help support kidney health.

Customizing for Individual Needs

Customizing dietary recommendations for individual needs is crucial for effectively preventing or managing kidney stones, as the underlying causes and risk factors can vary among individuals. Here's how to tailor dietary strategies to meet specific needs:

- **Personalized Nutrient Needs:** Consider individual nutrient requirements based on factors such as age, gender, weight, activity level, and medical history. Some individuals may have specific nutritional needs that require adjustments to their diet, such as those with certain medical conditions or dietary restrictions.

- **Identifying Specific Stone Types:** Determine the type of kidney stones a person is prone to forming, as dietary recommendations may vary depending on the composition of the stones. For example, individuals with calcium oxalate stones may need to limit high-oxalate foods, while those with uric acid stones may need to reduce purine-rich foods.

- **Assessing Risk Factors:** Evaluate individual risk factors for kidney stone formation, such as family history, medical conditions (e.g., obesity, diabetes), medications, and dietary habits. Customized dietary recommendations can help address specific risk factors and minimize the likelihood of stone recurrence.

- **Tailoring Hydration Needs:** Adjust fluid intake recommendations based on individual hydration needs, urine output, and activity level. Some individuals may require higher fluid intake to maintain adequate urine volume and prevent stone formation, while others may need to monitor fluid intake more closely due to medical conditions like kidney disease.

- **Adapting to Preferences and Lifestyle:** Consider personal preferences, cultural influences, and lifestyle factors when developing dietary recommendations. Customizing meal plans to include familiar foods and flavors can help improve adherence and long-term success.

- **Monitoring Progress:** Regularly monitor progress and adjust dietary recommendations as needed based on changes in kidney function, stone formation, or other health outcomes. Collaboration with healthcare professionals, such as nephrologists or registered dietitians, can provide valuable guidance and support throughout the process.

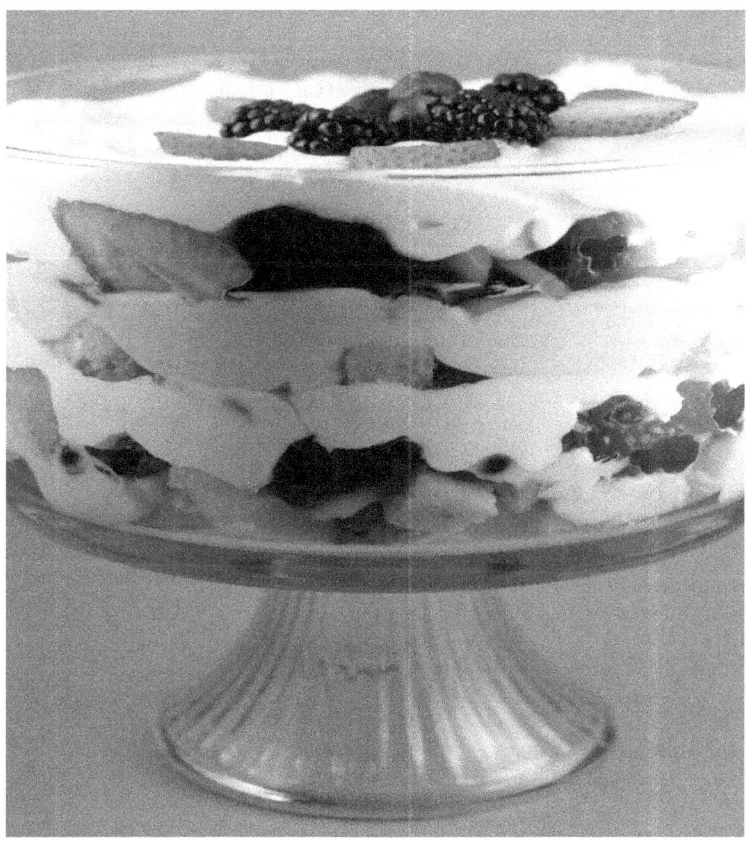

CHAPTER 9: CONCLUSION

Sustainable Lifestyle Changes

Implementing sustainable lifestyle changes is essential for preventing kidney stones and maintaining kidney health in the long term. Here are some strategies for making sustainable lifestyle changes to reduce the risk of kidney stones:

- **Hydration:** Stay consistently hydrated by drinking an adequate amount of water throughout the day. Aim to drink at least 8-10 cups of water daily, or more if you have a history of kidney stones or engage in strenuous physical activity. Keep a reusable water bottle with you as a reminder to stay hydrated wherever you go.

- **Balanced Diet:** Adopt a balanced diet that includes a variety of nutrient-dense foods, such as fruits, vegetables, whole grains, lean proteins, and healthy fats. Choose low-oxalate foods whenever possible and limit the intake of high-oxalate foods, sodium, and processed foods. Incorporate kidney stone-friendly recipes into your meal rotation to maintain dietary consistency.

- **Portion Control:** Practice portion control to avoid overeating and maintain a healthy weight. Use smaller plates and utensils to help control portion sizes, and be mindful of serving sizes when dining out or preparing meals at home. Pay attention to hunger and fullness cues to prevent overindulgence.

- **Regular Physical Activity:** Engage in regular physical activity to support overall health and reduce the risk of kidney stones. Aim for at least 150 minutes of moderate-intensity exercise or 75 minutes of vigorous-intensity exercise per week, along with muscle-strengthening activities on two or more days per week. Find activities you enjoy, such as walking, cycling, swimming, or yoga, and incorporate them into your routine.

- **Stress Management:** Practice stress-reducing techniques such as mindfulness, meditation, deep breathing exercises, or yoga to help manage stress levels. Chronic stress can contribute to dehydration and kidney stone formation, so finding healthy ways to cope with stress is essential for kidney health.

- **Regular Monitoring:** Stay proactive about monitoring your kidney health by scheduling regular check-ups with your healthcare provider. Discuss any concerns or changes in symptoms, and follow recommended guidelines for kidney stone prevention, including dietary modifications and medication management.

Celebrating Successes

- Celebrating successes, no matter how small, is crucial for maintaining motivation and momentum when preventing or managing kidney stones. Here are some ways to celebrate achievements and milestones along the journey:

- **Set Goals:** Establish clear, achievable goals related to kidney stone prevention or management, such as increasing water intake, following a low-oxalate diet, or maintaining a healthy weight. Celebrate each milestone reached, whether it's drinking a certain amount of water each day for a week or successfully sticking to a kidney stone-friendly meal plan.

- **Acknowledge Progress:** Take time to acknowledge and celebrate progress made toward your goals. Keep track of your achievements, whether it's reducing the frequency of kidney stone episodes, improving hydration levels, or adopting healthier lifestyle habits. Reflect on how far you've come and the positive changes you've made.

- **Reward Yourself:** Treat yourself to rewards or incentives as you reach key milestones in your kidney stone prevention journey. Choose rewards that align with your goals and promote overall health, such as purchasing a new reusable water bottle, enjoying a relaxing massage, or indulging in a healthy meal at your favorite restaurant.

- **Share Successes:** Share your successes with friends, family, or support groups who can offer encouragement and celebrate your achievements with you. Celebrating successes together creates a sense of community and reinforces positive behaviors and habits.

- **Practice Self-Care:** Incorporate self-care activities into your routine to reward yourself for your hard work and dedication.

Take time to relax and recharge with activities like meditation, yoga, a bubble bath, or a leisurely walk in nature. Self-care promotes overall well-being and helps maintain a positive mindset.

- **Stay Positive:** Focus on the positive aspects of your journey and celebrate the small victories along the way. Celebrating successes boosts morale, enhances motivation, and reinforces the importance of ongoing efforts to prevent kidney stones and prioritize kidney health.

Moving Forward with Kidney Health

Moving forward with kidney health involves a proactive approach to prevention, management, and overall well-being. Here are some key strategies to help you prioritize and maintain kidney health:

- **Commit to Healthy Habits:** Make a commitment to adopting and maintaining healthy lifestyle habits that support kidney health. This includes staying hydrated by drinking an adequate amount of water each day,

- following a balanced diet rich in fruits, vegetables, whole grains, lean proteins, and healthy fats, engaging in regular physical activity, managing stress effectively, and avoiding habits that can harm kidney function, such as smoking and excessive alcohol consumption.

- **Educate Yourself:** Take the time to educate yourself about kidney health, including risk factors for kidney stones, signs and symptoms of kidney problems, and strategies for prevention and management. Understanding your kidneys and how to care for them empowers you to make informed decisions and take proactive steps to protect and support kidney function.

- **Monitor Kidney Function:** Stay proactive about monitoring your kidney function by scheduling regular check-ups with your healthcare provider.
- Blood tests, urine tests, and imaging studies can help assess kidney function and identify any potential issues early on.

- Be proactive in discussing any concerns or changes in symptoms with your healthcare provider and follow their recommendations for follow-up care and management.

- **Manage Underlying Conditions:** If you have underlying medical conditions that can affect kidney health, such as diabetes, hypertension, or obesity, work closely with your healthcare provider to manage these conditions effectively.

- Keeping these conditions under control can help reduce the risk of kidney complications and promote overall kidney health.

- **Stay Hydrated:** Proper hydration is essential for kidney health, as it helps flush out toxins and waste products from the body and prevents the formation of kidney stones. Drink plenty of water throughout the day, especially in hot weather or when engaging in physical activity. Monitor your urine color as a simple way to gauge hydration status – aim for pale yellow urine, indicating adequate hydration.

- **Practice Medication Safety:** Be mindful of the medications you take and their potential impact on kidney health. Some medications, including over-the-counter pain relievers like nonsteroidal anti-inflammatory drugs (NSAIDs) and certain antibiotics, can harm kidney function if used excessively or inappropriately. Always follow your healthcare provider's instructions when taking medications and avoid self-medicating without professional guidance.

- **Seek Support:** Surround yourself with a supportive network of friends, family, and healthcare professionals who can offer encouragement, guidance, and assistance as you prioritize kidney health. Joining support groups or online communities can also provide valuable resources, information, and camaraderie with others who share similar experiences and goals.

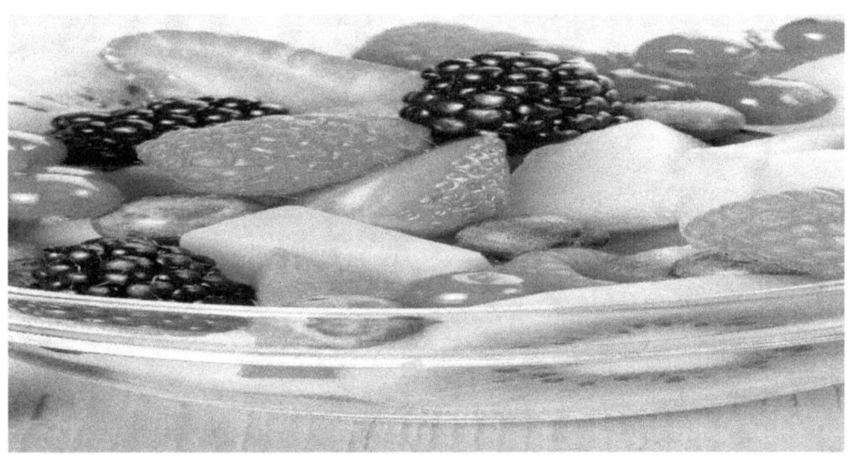

www.ingramcontent.com/pod-product-compliance
Lightning Source LLC
Chambersburg PA
CBHW070810260726
48660CB00005B/1800